Kidney Cancer. Recent Results of Basic and Clinical Research

Contributions to Nephrology

Vol. 128

Series Editors *G.M. Berlyne*, Beersheva, Brooklyn, N.Y.
C. Ronco, Vicenza

KARGER

Basel · Freiburg · Paris · London · New York ·
New Delhi · Bangkok · Singapore · Tokyo · Sydney

Kidney Cancer

Recent Results of Basic and Clinical Research

Volume Editor *O. Hino*, Tokyo

45 figures, 6 in color, and 10 tables, 1999

KARGER

Basel · Freiburg · Paris · London · New York ·
New Delhi · Bangkok · Singapore · Tokyo · Sydney

Okio Hino
Department of Experimental Pathology
Cancer Institute
1-37-1 Kami-Ikebukuro
Toshima-ku, Tokyo 170-8455 (Japan)

Library of Congress Cataloging-in-Publication Data
Kidney cancer / volume editor, Hino, O.
(Contributions to nephrology; vol. 128)
Includes bibliographical references and index.
1. Kidneys – Cancer. I. Hino, Okio. II. Contributions to nephrology; v. 128
[DNLM: 1. Kidney Neoplasms. WJ 358 K46 1999]
RC280, K5 K526 1999 616.99′461 – dc21
ISBN 3-8055-6919-X

Bibliographic Indices. This publication is listed in bibliographic services, including Current Contents® and Index Medicus.

Drug Dosage. The authors and the publisher have exerted every effort to ensure that drug selection and dosage set forth in this text are in accord with current recommendations and practice at the time of publication. However, in view of ongoing research, changes in government regulations, and the constant flow of information relating to drug therapy and drug reactions, the reader is urged to check the package insert for each drug for any change in indications and dosage and for added warnings and precautions. This is particularly important when the recommended agent is a new and/or infrequently employed drug.

www.karger.com
Printed in Switzerland on acid-free paper by Reinhardt Druck, Basel
ISBN 3–8055–6919–X

Contents

Preface

Cancer is a heritable disorder of somatic cells and gene expression disease. Environment and heredity both operate in the origin of human cancer. Recently the responsible genes of familial kidney cancer syndromes were cloned and identified: von Hippel-Lindau disease (VHL gene on human 3p25, autosomal dominant); papillary renal cell carcinoma (MET proto-oncogene on human 7q31, autosomal dominant); tuberous sclerosis (TSC1 and TSC2 genes on human 9q34 and 16p13.3, respectively; autosomal dominant), and Wilms' tumor (WT1 gene on human 11p13, autosomal dominant).

Hereditary kidney cancer should prove valuable in understanding the mechanisms of disease and the development of therapeutic treatments.

This book brings together some of the most recent advances made in kidney cancers. Leading investigators present recent results including VHL, MET, TSC1 and TSC2, WT1 genes, as well as environmentally induced kidney cancers (long-term hemodialysis and chemically induced renal cell carcinomas) and therapeutic treatments (surgery and gene therapy), providing an excellent survey of this field.

Hino O (ed): Kidney Cancer. Recent Results of Basic and Clinical Research.
Contrib Nephrol. Basel, Karger, 1999, vol 128, pp 1–10

Germline and Somatic Mutations in von Hippel-Lindau Disease Gene and Its Significance in the Development of Kidney Cancer

Taro Shuin[a], *Keiichi Kondo*[b], *Shingo Ashida*[a], *Heiwa Okuda*[a], *Minoru Yoshida*[b], *Hiroshi Kanno*[c], *Masahiro Yao*[b]

[a] Department of Urology, Kochi Medical School, Kochi, and Departments of [b] Urology and [c] Neurosurgery, Yokohama City University School of Medicine, Yokohama City, Japan

Introduction

The von Hippel-Lindau (VHL) disease gene is a putative tumor-suppressor gene responsible for VHL disease, an autosomal dominantly inherited multitumor syndrome. The VHL-associated tumors and cysts include retinal angioma (RA), central nervous system (CNS) hemangioblastomas (HBs), renal cell carcinoma (RCC), pheochromocytoma (pheo), neuroendocrine tumors in the pancreas, and cysts in the kidney, pancreas, inner ear, epididymis and female reproductive organs. Clear cell RCC is a major risk of death in VHL disease [1]. The average age at the development of the kidney cancer in the VHL patients is 39.

The gene responsible for VHL disease was isolated by positional cloning at 3p25–26 by Latif et al. [2] in 1993. The isolated cDNA encodes 639 nucleotides (213 amino acids) in 3 exons as the coding region (fig. 1). The open reading frame has 2 start sites. The encoded proteins from the first or second start site are 24 and 19 kD, respectively. The 24-kD protein that actually migrates 30 kD in SDS gel is localized mainly in the cytosol and to a lesser degree in the nucleus. The 19-kD protein is equally distributed in the cytosol and nucleus [3–6]. It has specific acidic pentamer repeats at the top of exon 1 that has 48% homology with trypanozoma brucei (fig. 1).

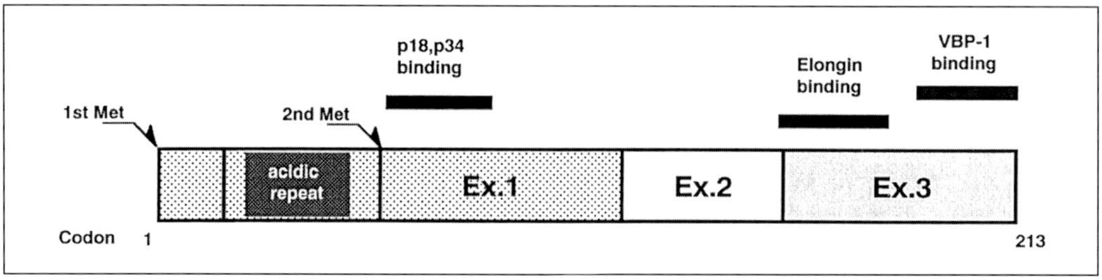

Fig. 1. Three exons of the VHL gene and the binding regions of VHL-binding proteins.

Table 1. Classification of VHL disease

Type	RA	HB	RCC	PHEO
VHL type 1	+	+	+	–
VHL type 2A	+	+	–	+
VHL type 2B	+	+	+	+

RA = Retinal angioma; HB = central nervous system hemangioblastoma; RCC = renal cell carcinoma; PHEO = pheochrocytoma.

Loss of function in the VHL protein (pVHL) is also responsible for the development of sporadic types of VHL-associated tumors, such as sporadic clear cell RCC, RA, CNS HBs, and a minority of pheos and gliomas [7–11].

VHL diseases without pheos and those with pheos are classified as type 1 or type 2, respectively. Type-2 VHL disease is subdivided into 2A and 2B without or with RCC (table 1). The molecular genetic characterization of the germline and sporadic types of VHL-associated tumors was a major step towards understanding the molecular pathogenesis of VHL disease and RCC.

The detection of mutations in the VHL gene promotes accurate presymptomatic diagnosis within VHL kindreds. Genetic testing encourages early detection of presymptomatic carrier germline mutation. It also avoids unnecessary medical examination for noncarriers of the germline mutation.

Previous studies revealed several binding proteins for pVHL and its associated functions. These are Elongin B, C and Cul2, VBP1, SP1, some species of protein kinase C (PKC), and fibronectin [12–16]. pVHL complexes with Elongin B, C and Cul2. Cul2 has homology to yeast CDC53 [13]. The complex of pVHL, Elongin B, C and Cul2 decreases the half life of hypoxia-inducible mRNAs, such as vascular endothelial growth factor, glucose transporter 1,

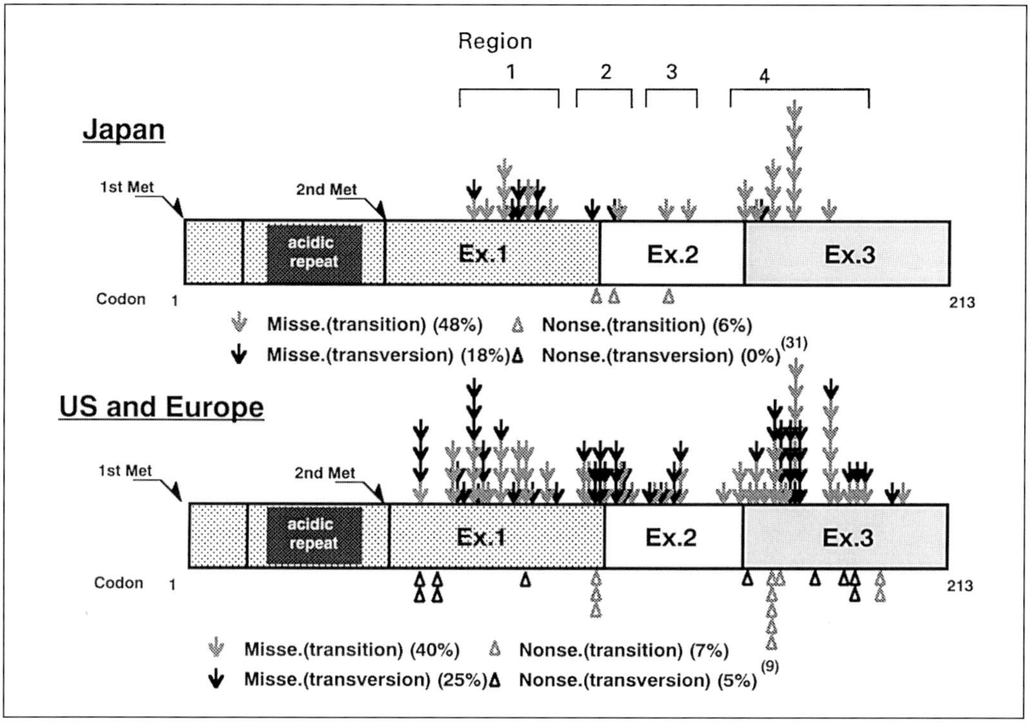

Fig. 2. Germline missense or nonsense mutation plotted on the 3 exons of VHL gene. Black arrows denote missense mutations with base transversion. Gray arrows denotes missense mutations with base transition. Black arrowheads denote missense mutations of base transversion. Gray arrowheads denote missense mutations with base transition.

and platelet-derived growth factor β chain [17]. pVHL also binds fibronectin at its top and end [18]. It is supposed to help to make proper conformation of fibronectin in the Golgi apparatus. pVHL works for the cellular export and appropriate distribution of fibronectin in the extracellular matrix.

Most of the tumors in VHL disease and its sporadic type tumors have similar pathological characteristics. RA, CNS HB, and clear cell RCC have an abundant vascular structure and clear cytoplasm that are explained by the loss of Elongin complex formation with mutated pVHL. Only pheos that are observed in VHL type-2 disease, do not have such a pathological appearance. This suggests that mutated pVHL in VHL type 2 has other unknown biological functions.

Here we plotted published germline and somatic mutations on 3 exons of the VHL gene [7, 19–28] (fig. 2–5). In so doing we have been able to describe some characteristic features in the germline mutation and those in the somatic mutation of the VHL gene in sporadic RCCs. Japanese results are compared with those of Western countries in both germline and somatic missense mutations to examine racial differences.

Characteristics of the Germline Mutations of the VHL Gene

Germline mutations include missense or nonsense mutations, deletions, insertions, hypermethylations or rearrangements in a larger scale of DNA detected by Southern blot or pulse field gel electrophoresis, or fluorescent in situ hybridization. Technical progress has increased the detection rate of mutations up to 100% [29]. According to the previous publications for germline and somatic mutations of the VHL gene together with our unpublished results, we plotted missense or nonsense mutations, deletions and insertions on the 3 exons of the VHL gene [7, 19–28] (fig. 2, 3). The incidences of some types of mutation in VHL disease are critically different from those in sporadic RCCs that have been well examined for VHL gene mutations. Missense mutations in VHL disease are more frequent than in sporadic RCC. In Japan and both the US and Europe, it is 66%. Missense mutations clustered in 4 regions of the VHL gene in Japan and the US and Europe together. They are located the second half of exon 1, the boundary of exons 1 and 2, the middle portion of exon 2, and the top portion of exon 3 which corresponds to the Elongin B-C binding domain (fig. 2). Mutations are not detected in the acidic pentamer repeats in exon 1. Mutations in the boundary of exons 1 and 2 and the middle portion of exon 2 are not as frequent in Japan as in the US and Europe. The biological consequence of mutations around the top portion of exon 3 is considered as the loss of binding of Elongin B, C, Cul2 to pVHL and increased stability of hypoxia-inducible mRNAs. The mutations clustered in the boundary of exons 1 and 2 might correspond to the PKC-binding domain. The biological consequences of this mutation could be loss of binding of PKC from VHL and a subsequent gain in function of PKC. Mutations at Tyr98His (VHL type 2A) or Tyr112His (VHL type 2A) are close to this region. Type-2A VHL diseases are observed in the Black Forest in Germany and Pennsylvania in the US, and often develop HB, RA and pheos [23]. However, they have a low risk of RCC development in the kidney. At present, there is no clear biological meaning for the cluster of the missense mutations in the second half of exon 1 (fig. 1, Region 1). Some of this region corresponds to the p18 and p34 binding domain [30]. A deletion or insertion mutation is detected in less than 22% of germline cases. There is no characteristic feature in the sites of nonsense mutation, insertion or deletion in germline cases both in Japan and the US

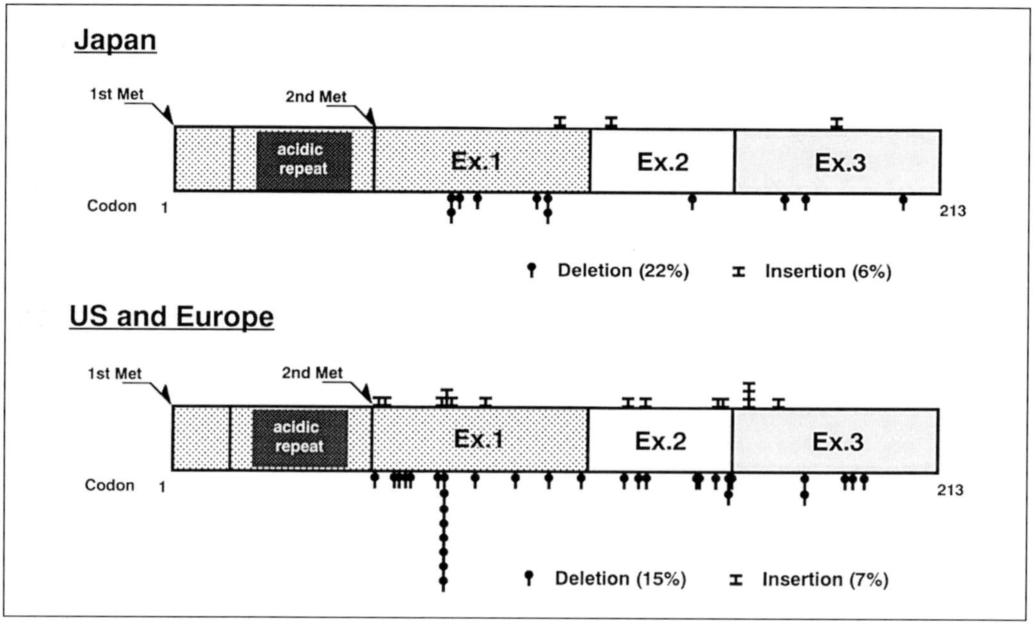

Fig. 3. Germline deletions or insertions plotted on the VHL gene.

and Europe together, except one accumulation deletions in the second half of exon 1. They probably result in the loss of function of pVHL (fig. 3).

When base changes in the germline missense mutation in Japan is compared with those in the US and Europe, the incidence of base transition is more frequent in Japan than in the US and Europe, especially in the mutations around the Elongin B-C binding domain (fig. 2, Region 4, 13/14 versus 20/36). This suggests that a different genetic mechanism for germline mutation is present in Japan.

Characteristics of the Somatic Mutation of the VHL Gene in Sporadic Clear Cell RCCs

Somatic mutations in the VHL gene are detected only in clear cell RCCs. No other pathological type of RCC exhibits the VHL gene mutation. A somatic mutation in the VHL gene in clear cell RCC is characterized by the high incidence of deletion or insertion mutations. It results in the truncation of pVHL. It also causes a shorter half-life of pVHL (unpubl. data). Thus, even if some function remains in the truncated protein, it hardly works. One hundred and two somatic mutations in Japan consisted of 49 deletions (including 1

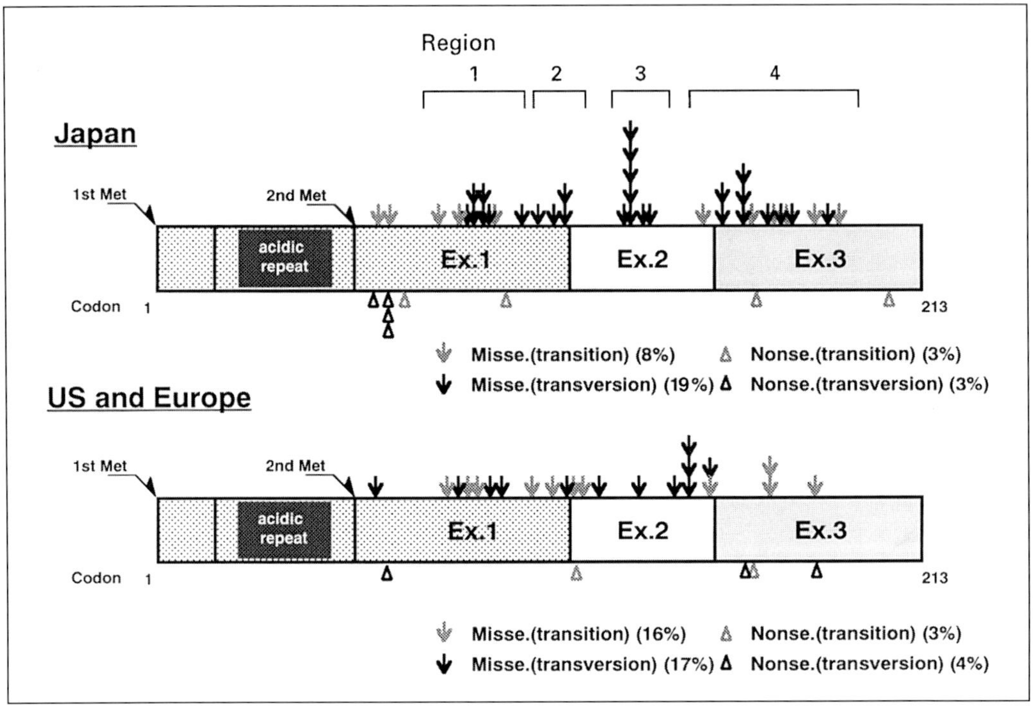

Fig. 4. Somatic missense or nonsense mutations of RCCs plotted on the VHL gene. Black arrows denotes missense mutations of base transversion. Gray arrows denote missense mutations with base transition. Black arrowheads denote missense mutations of base transversion. Gray arrowheads denote missense mutations with base transition.

splice-site mutation), 18 insertions, 7 nonsense and 28 missense mutations. Thus, 75% of the mutations (deletion, insertion, nonsense, and splice-site mutations) result in truncation of the VHL protein [31]. Those in the US and Europe have similar features. The function of pVHL will be lost in most tumors. Mutations of the VHL gene are observed in 53% of sporadic clear cell RCCs, close to 20% of cases showing hypermethylation in the CpG island of the promoter region in the VHL gene in the literature [32]. Therefore, less than 30% of the sporadic clear cell RCCs have other initiating genetic events for tumor development. Deletion or insertion mutations do not have a clustered region in sporadic clear cell RCCs. We compared missense mutations of sporadic RCC with germline cases. Although it is less apparent, similar clustered regions are observed (fig. 4). Missense mutations are distributed in the second half of exon 1, the boundary of exons 1 and 2, the middle portion of exon 2, and the top portion of exon 3 corresponding to the Elongin B, C,

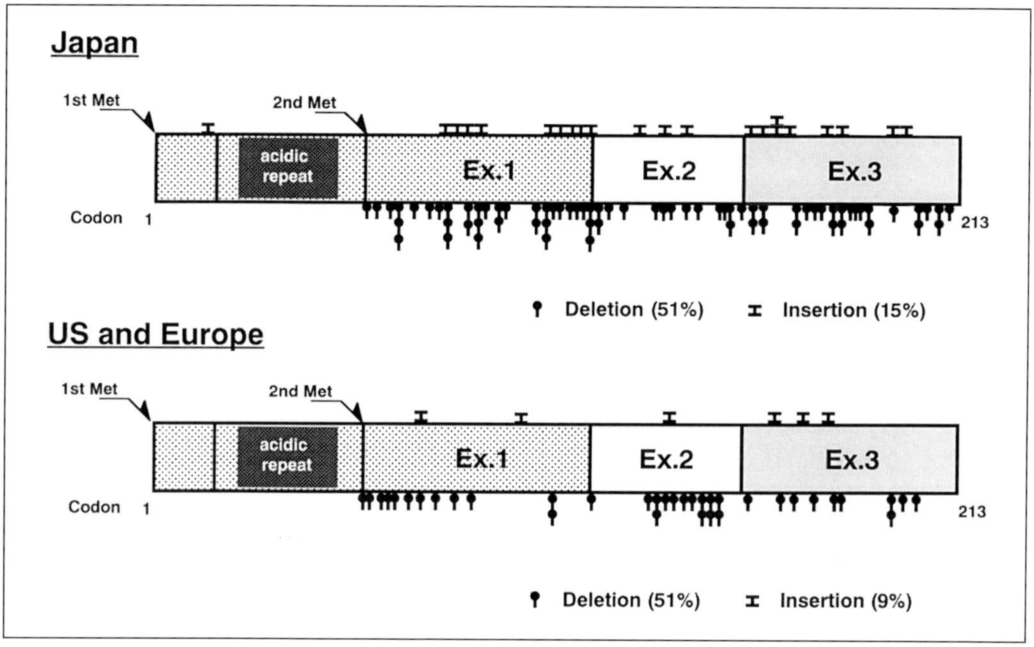

Fig. 5. Somatic insertions and deletions of RCCs plotted on the 3 exons of the VHL gene.

and Cul2 binding domain. This suggests that sporadic RCCs with missense mutations develop through genetic events similar to germline tumors with missense mutations. When clinical or pathological characteristics are analyzed in these sporadic clear cell RCCs, mutations in sporadic tumors are observed to a similar frequency in all clinical stages (43–58%) and pathological grades (46–63%) [31]. This finding suggests that mutations in the VHL gene occur in early stages, probably in the initiative stage in the carcinogenesis of clear cell RCC.

Chromosomal (3;8) translocations in familial RCC cases have suggested other possible tumor-suppressor genes in the initiation of kidney cancers. However, families with this translocation also show mutations in the VHL gene [7]. Therefore, the VHL tumor-suppressor gene is the major gene responsible for the development of most sporadic RCCs.

Summary and Future Aspect

Here, we show several features of the germline mutation in the VHL gene and somatic mutation of sporadic clear cell RCCs.

Germline mutations in the VHL gene have been thoroughly examined in Japan and the US and Europe. Germline mutations in the VHL gene are characterized by a high frequency of missense mutations in all countries. Most type-2 VHL show missense mutations. VHL type 1 also has a high frequency of missense mutations. The missense mutations have 4 clustered regions in the VHL gene.

Sporadic human RCCs have also been well examined for somatic mutations in the VHL gene. Although all types of mutation, including hypermethylation of the VHL gene, have been detected, somatic mutation of the VHL gene in sporadic RCC is characterized by a high frequency of deletion or insertion mutation. This is in contrast to germline cases. Deletion or insertion mutation of sporadic RCC in the VHL gene has no specific feature both in Japan and Western countries. Although it is less apparent, missense mutation of the VHL gene in sporadic clear cell RCCs shows clustered regions similar to those in germline mutation. Germline mutation of the VHL gene is a different event from somatic mutation of the VHL that occurs only in limited types of organs, probably by carcinogens. However, current results suggest that the origin of germline and somatic missense mutations may share a similar genetic mechanism.

Exceptional cases are mutations at Tyr98His (VHL type 2A) or Tyr112His (VHL type 2A) that are observed in the VHL type2A, which has a low risk of RCC. This mutated pVHL may have a different function for tumorigenesis of pheos.

Recent molecular biological work has revealed several interesting biological functions in the VHL gene. Some of them are based on studies of germline and somatic mutation. Some functions of the VHL gene remain unknown. When these functions are more precisely identified, there will be further progress in the diagnosis, treatment and prevention of VHL-associated tumors and their sporadic types of tumors.

Note Added in Proof

After preparation of this manuscript, Stebbins et al. [33] showed the structure of VHL-Elongin BC complex. It revealed β-sheet domain (amino acid 63 to 154) in the N-terminal portion of VHL and α-helix (amino acid 155 to 192) in the C-terminal portion. β-Domain, that may correspond to region 1 to 3, is supposed to have unknown binding proteins.

References

1 Maher ER, Yates RW, Harries R, Benjamin C, Harris R, Moore AT, Ferguson-Smith MA: Clinical features and natural history of von Hippel-Lindau disease. Q J Med 1990;77:1151–1163.

2 Latif F, Tory K, Gnarra J, Yao M, Duh FM, Orcutt ML, Stackhouse T, Kuzmin I, Modi W, Geil L, Schmidt L, Zhou F, Li H, Wei MH, Chen F, Glenn G, Choyke P, Walther MM, Weng Y, Duan DR, Dean M, Glavac D, Richards FM, Crossey PA, Ferguson-Smith MA, Paslier DL, Chumakov I, Cohen D, Chinault C, Maher ER, Linehan VM, Zbar B, Lerman MI: Identification of the von Hippel-Lindau disease tumor suppressor gene. Science 1993;260:1317–1320.

3 Duan DR, Humphrey JS, Chen DY, Weng Y, Sukegawa J, Lee S, Gnarra JR, Linehan WM: Characterization of the VHL tumor suppressor gene product: Localization, complex formation, and the effect of natural inactivating mutations. Proc Natl Acad Sci USA 1995;92:6459–6463.

4 Lee S, Chen DY, Humphrey JS, Gnarra JR, Linehan WM, Klausner RD: Nuclear/cytoplasmic localization of the von Hippel-Lindau tumor suppressor gene product is determined by cell density. Proc Natl Acad Sci USA 1996;93:1770–1775.

5 Iliopoulos O, Ohh M, Kaelin WG Jr: pVHL19 is a biologically active product of the von Hippel-Lindau gene arising from internal translation initiation. Proc Natl Acad Sci USA 1998;95:11661–11666.

6 Schoenfeld A, Davidowitz EJ, Burk RD: A second major native von Hippel-Lindau gene product, initiated from an internal translation start site, functions as a tumor suppressor. Proc Natl Acad Sci USA 1998;95:8817–8822.

7 Gnarra JR, Tory K, Weng Y, Schmidt L, Wei MH, Li H, Latif F, Liu S, Chen F, Duh FM, Lubensky I, Duan DR, Florence C, Pozzatti R, Walther MM, Bander NH, Grossman HB, Brauch H, Pomer S, Brooks JD, Isaacs WB, Lerman MI, Zbar B, Linehan WM: Mutations of the VHL tumour suppressor gene in renal carcinoma. Nat Genet 1994;7:85–90.

8 Shuin T, Kondo K, Torigoe S, Kishida T, Kubota Y, Hosaka M, Nagashima Y, Kitamura H, Latif F, Zbar B, Lerman MI, Yao M: Frequent somatic mutations and loss of heterozygosity of the von Hippel-Lindau tumor suppressor gene in primary human renal cell carcinomas. Cancer Res 1994; 54:2852–2855.

9 Kanno H, Kondo K, Ito S, Yamamoto I, Fujii S, Torigoe S, Sakai N, Hosaka M, Shuin T, Yao M: Somatic mutations of the von Hippel-Lindau tumor suppressor gene in sporadic central nervous system hemangioblastomas. Cancer Res 1994;54:4845–4847.

10 Eng C, Crossey PA, Mulligan LM, Healey CS, Houghton C, Prowse A, Chew SL, Dahia PL, O'Riordan JL, Toledo SP, Smith DP, Maher ER, Ponder EAJ: Mutations in the RET proto-oncogene and the von Hippel-Lindau disease tumour suppressor gene in sporadic and syndromic phaeochromocytomas. J Med Genet 1995;32:934–937.

11 Kanno H, Shuin T, Kondo K, Yamamoto I, Ito S, Shinonaga M, Yoshida M, Yao M: Somatic mutations of the von Hippel-Lindau tumor suppressor gene and loss of heterozygosity on chromosome 3p in human glial tumors. Cancer Res 1997;57:1035–1038.

12 Duan DR, Pause A, Burgess WH, Aso T, Chen DY, Garrett KP, Conaway RC, Conaway JW, Linehan WM, Klausner RD: Inhibition of transcription elongation by the VHL tumor suppressor protein. Science 1995;269:1402–1406.

13 Lonergan KM, Iliopoulos O, Ohh M, Kamura T, Conaway RC, Conaway JW, Kaelin WG Jr: Regulation of hypoxia-inducible mRNAs by the von Hippel-Lindau tumor suppressor protein requires binding to complexes containing elongins B/C and Cul2. Mol Cell Biol 1998;18:732–741.

14 Tsuchiya H, Iseda T, Hino O: Identification of a novel protein (VBP-1) binding to the von Hippel-Lindau (VHL) tumor suppressor gene product. Cancer Res 1996;56:2881–2885.

15 Mukhopadhyay D, Knebelmann B, Cohen HT, Ananth S, Sukhatme VP: The von Hippel-Lindau tumor suppressor gene product interacts with Sp1 to repress vascular endothelial growth factor promoter activity. Mol Cell Biol 1997;17:5629–5639.

16 Pal S, Claffey KP, Dvorak HF, Mukhopadhyay D: The von Hippel-Lindau gene product inhibits vascular permeability factor/vascular endothelial growth factor expression in renal cell carcinoma by blocking protein kinase C pathways. J Biol Chem 1997;272:27509–27512.

17 Kaelin WG, Iliopoulos O, Lonergan KM, Ohh M: Functions of the von Hippel-Lindau tumour suppressor protein. J Intern Med 1998;243:535–539.

18 Ohh M, Yauch RL, Lonergan KM, Whaley JM, Stemmer-Rachamimov AO, Louis DN, Gavin BJ, Kley N, Kaelin WG Jr, Iliopoulos O: The von Hippel-Lindau tumor suppressor protein is required for proper assembly of an extracellular fibronectin matrix. Mol Cell 1998;1:959–968.
19 Whaley JM, Naglich J, Gelbert L, Hsia YE, Lamiell JM, Green JS, Collins D, Neumann HPH, Laidlaw J, Li FP, Klein-Szanto AJP, Seizinger BR, Kley N: Germ-line mutations in the von Hippel-Lindau tumor-suppressor gene are similar to somatic von Hippel-Lindau aberrations in sporadic renal cell carcinoma. Am J Hum Genet 1994;55:1092–1102.
20 Foster K, Prowse A, van den Berg A, Fleming S, Hulsbeek MM, Crossey PA, Richards FM, Cairns P, Affara NA, Ferguson-Smith MA, Buys C, Maher ER: Somatic mutations of the von Hippel-Lindau disease tumour suppressor gene in non-familial clear cell renal carcinoma. Hum Mol Genet 1994;3:2169–2173.
21 Brauch H, Kishida T, Glavac D, Chen F, Pausch F, Hofler H, Latif F, Lerman MI, Zbar B, Neumann HP: Von Hippel-Lindau (VHL) disease with pheochromocytoma in the Black Forest region of Germany: Evidence for a founder effect. Hum Genet 1995;95:551–556.
22 Bailly M, Bain C, Favrot MC, Ozturk M: Somatic mutations of Von Hippel-Lindau (VHL) tumor-suppressor gene in European kidney cancers. Int J Cancer 1995;63:660–664.
23 Zbar B, Kishida T, Chen F, Schmidt L, Maher ER, Richards FM, Crossey PA, Webster AR, Affara NA, Ferguson-Smith MA, Brauch H, Glavac D, Neumann HP, Tisherman S, Mulvihill JJ, Gross DJ, Shuin T, Whaley J, Seizinger B, Kley N, Olschwang S, Boisson C, Richard S, Lips CHM, Linehan WM, Lerman M: Germline mutations in the Von Hippel-Lindau disease (VHL) gene in families from North America, Europe, and Japan. Hum Mutat 1996;8:348–357.
24 Crossey PA, Richards FM, Foster K, Green JS, Prowse A, Latif F, Lerman MI, Zbar B, Affara NA, Ferguson-Smith MA, et al: Identification of intragenic mutations in the von Hippel-Lindau disease tumour suppressor gene and correlation with disease phenotype. Hum Mol Genet 1994;3: 1303–1308.
25 Chen F, Kishida T, Yao M, Hustad T, Glavac D, Dean M, Gnarra JR, Orcutt ML, Duh FM, Glenn G, Green J, Hsia YE, Lamiell J, Li H, Wei MH, Schmidt L, Tory K, Kuzmin I, Stackhouse T, Latif F, Linehan WM, Lerman M, Zbar B: Germline mutations in the von Hippel-Lindau disease tumor suppressor gene: Correlations wih phenotype. Hum Mutat 1995;5:66–75.
26 Kanno H, Shuin T, Kondo K, Ito S, Hosaka M, Torigoe S, Fujii S, Tanaka Y, Yamamoto I, Kim I, Yao M: Molecular genetic diagnosis of von Hippel-Lindau disease: Analysis of five Japanese families. Jpn J Cancer Res 1996;87:423–428.
27 Clinical Research Group for VHL in Japan: Germline mutations in the von Hippel-Lindau disease (VHL) gene in Japanese VHL. Hum Mol Genet 1995;4:2233–2237.
28 Suzuki H, Ueda T, Komiya A, Okano T, Isaka S, Shimazaki J, Ito H: Mutational state of von Hippel Lindau and adenomatous polyposis coli genes in renal tumors. Oncology 1997;54:252–257.
29 Stolle C, Glenn G, Zbar B, Humphrey JS, Choyke P, Walther M, Pack S, Hurley K, Andrey C, Klausner R, Linehan WM: Improved detection of germline mutations in the von Hippel-Lindau disease tumor suppressor gene. Hum Mutat 1998;12:417–423.
30 Kishida T, Stackhouse TM, Chen F, Lerman MI, Zbar B: Cellular proteins that bind the von Hippel-Lindau disease gene product: Mapping of binding domains and the effect of missense mutations. Cancer Res 1995;55:4544–4548.
31 Yao M, Kondo K, Yoshida M, Kishida T, Shuin T: Molecular genetics of the kidney cancers: Implication of the VHL tumor suppressor gene; in Niimura M, Otsuka F, Hino O (eds): Gann Monograph on Cancer Research. Japan Scientific Societies Press, Tokyo, 1999, pp 205–214.
32 Herman JG, Latif F, Weng Y, Lerman MI, Zbar B, Liu S, Samid D, Duan DS, Gnarra JR, Linehan WM, et al: Silencing of the VHL tumor-suppressor gene by DNA methylation in renal carcinoma. Proc Natl Acad Sci USA 1994;91:9700–9704.
33 Stebbins CE, Kaelin WG Jr, Pavletich NP: Structures of the VHL-Elongin C-Elongin B complex: Implications for VHL tumor suppressor function. Science 1999;284:455–460.

Taro Shuin, MD, Department of Urology, Kochi Medical School, Kochi (Japan)
Tel. +81 888 80 2401, Fax +81 888 80 2404

Hino O (ed): Kidney Cancer. Recent Results of Basic and Clinical Research.
Contrib Nephrol. Basel, Karger, 1999, vol 128, pp 11–27

Hereditary Papillary Renal Carcinoma: Pathology and Pathogenesis

Laura Schmidt[a], *Irina Lubensky*[b], *W.M. Linehan*[c], *Berton Zbar*[d]

[a] Intramural Research Support Program, SAIC Frederick, National Cancer Institute-Frederick Cancer Research and Development Center, Frederick, Md.
[b] Laboratory of Pathology, National Institutes of Health, Bethesda, Md.
[c] Urologic Oncology Branch, National Institutes of Health, Bethesda, Md., and
[d] Laboratory of Immunobiology, National Cancer Institute-Frederick Cancer Research and Development Center, Frederick, Md., USA

Introduction

Papillary renal carcinomas (PRCs) comprise 10% of all tumors of the kidney [1]. PRCs are defined as renal carcinomas showing at least 75% papillary architecture [2]. Thoenes et al. [1], in their landmark studies of renal tumor pathology, recognized papillary (chromophil) renal carcinoma as an independent entity, and divided PRC into basophilic, eosinophilic and mixed subtypes. Recently, Delahunt and Eble [3] suggested that PRCs be divided into type 1 and type 2, which correspond respectively to the chromophil basophilic and chromophil eosinophilic subtypes of Thoenes et al. [1]. In general, PRC type 1 is characterized by the presence of short papillae lined by small epithelial cells with small, low-grade basophilic nuclei and scant amphophilic cytoplasm. PRC type 2 is characterized by papillae lined by large epithelial cells with high-grade nuclei and abundant eosinophilic cytoplasm.

Recently, Jiang et al. [4], and Amin et al. [5] compared the clinical characteristics of PRC types 1 and 2, and found evidence supporting the classification of PRCs suggested by Delahunt and Eble [3]. Jiang et al. [4] identified 52 PRCs among 615 renal tumors from the archives of the University of Basel. They selected for study 25 consecutive papillary renal tumors diagnosed after 1985 and before 1996. There were 9 type 1 and 16 type 2 tumors. Type 2 tumors were significantly larger, had a higher tumor stage, and higher nuclear

Table 1. Summary of MET proto-oncogene mutations in papillary renal carcinoma

DNA No.	Exon	Mutation	Codon
Somatic			
5458	16	C3528T	H1112Y
6052	16	C3564G	H1124D
6134	16	A3529T	H1112L
5468	18	C3831G	L1213V
4768	19	G3930C	D1246H
4769	19	T3936C	Y1248H
6046	19	A3937G	Y1248C
5422, 5434	19	T3997C	M1268T
Germline			
5946, 5274, 6088	16	G3522A	V1110I
6285	16	C3528T	H1112Y
5161, 4599, 5976	16	A3529G	H1112R
4374, 4762	17	T3640C	M1149T
5269	18	G3810T	V1206L
5243, 6067	19	G3906A	V1238I
5928	19	G3930A	D1246N
6059	19	T3936G	Y1248D
5456	19	A3937G	Y1248C
6082	19	T3997C	M1268T

From Schmidt et al. [11].

grade than type 1 PRCs. There were gains of chromosome 7 and 17 in 100% of type 1, but only 31% of type 2 had gains of 7p and 38% of type 2 had gains of 17p. Most type 1 tumors were stage pT1–2, and nuclear grade 1–2. Type 1 papillary renal tumors had a better prognosis ($p=0.03$) than type 2 tumors. No patient with PRC type 1 died of the disease. The authors suggested that type 1 and type 2 PRCs were two different entities, not the same tumor at different stages of evolution.

Zbar et al. [6–8] have described an inherited form of PRC. Affected family members developed multiple, bilateral PRCs. This disorder, designated hereditary papillary renal carcinoma (HPRC), was a consequence of missense mutations in the tyrosine kinase domain of the MET proto-oncogene (table 1; fig. 1). Mutations in the MET proto-oncogene were found in the germline of 6 of 7 HPRC families studied and in the tumors of 13% of PRC patients without a family history of renal malignancy [9–11].

Pathology of Renal Tumors in HPRC

MET mutation-positive PRCs were genetically and histologically different from renal tumors seen in other hereditary renal syndromes (von Hippel-Lindau [VHL] and familial renal oncocytoma) and from most sporadic renal tumors with prominent papillary architecture (PRC type 2, PRC with chromosome X;1 translocation, collecting duct carcinoma, conventional (clear) renal cell carcinoma (RCC) and metanephric adenoma). Patients with HPRC and germline MET mutations developed a spectrum of multiple, bilateral renal lesions with papillary histology: microscopic papillary lesions (<0.5 mm in size); papillary adenomas (<0.5 cm in size), and PRCs (>0.5 cm in size). HPRCs and sporadic PRCs with somatic MET mutations showed a distinctive PRC type 1 (chromophil basophilic carcinoma) histologic appearance (Lubensky et al., unpubl. data). Multiple microscopic renal lesions were common in kidneys of HPRC patients. These lesions had the same architecture and histology as papillary adenomas and PRC type 1.

The histopathology of archival papillary renal tumors and metastases in patients from 6 HPRC families with germline MET mutations and PRCs with somatic MET mutations from patients with no family history of renal tumors was evaluated (Lubensky et al., unpubl. data). All tumors were 75–100% papillary/tubulopapillary in architecture with slender, short papillae and delicate fibrovascular cores. The tumor papillae were lined by a single layer of small cells with small basophilic nuclei and inconspicuous amphophilic cytoplasm. Areas of 'clear' cells were common in HPRCs regardless of size and were seen in all renal tumors from HPRC patients. Like 'clear' cells of the conventional (clear) cell RCC, 'clear' cells in PRCs contained intracytoplasmic lipid and glycogen demonstrated by electron microscopy. However, unlike conventional (clear) cell RCC, 'clear' cells of PRCs had small basophilic nuclei and tumor areas composed of 'clear' cells lacked a fine vascular network. Foamy macrophages in fibrovascular cores, psammoma bodies, areas of hemorrhage and necrosis were common in HPRCs. Fibrous pseudocapsule was a common feature of PRCs >0.7 cm, but absent in smaller lesions. Fuhrman nuclear grade 1–2 (low grade) predominated in all papillary renal carcinomas with MET mutations but focal areas of Fuhrman nuclear grade 3 were seen in several tumors. Despite the low nuclear grade, 4 of 29 HPRC patients in the study had metastases to the lymph nodes, skeletal muscle and/or lungs (Lubensky et al., unpubl. data).

In summary, papillary renal neoplasms from the members of different HPRC families and from sporadic PRC patients with MET mutations share the same histological features of PRC type 1 (chromophil basophilic renal carcinoma). These results support the concept of genetic heterogeneity of

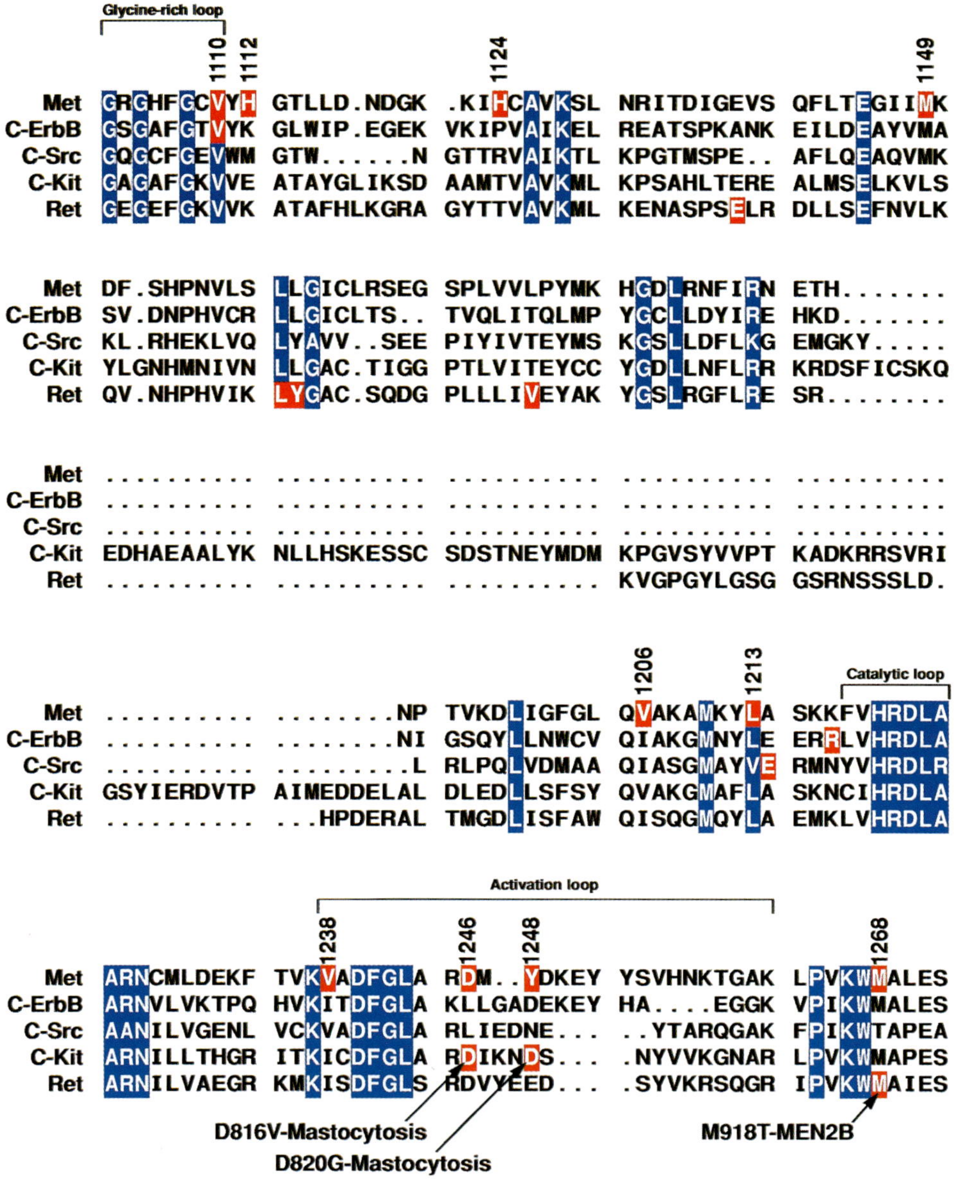
Glycine-rich loop
1110
1112
1124
1149
Met GRGHFGCVYH GTLLD.NDGK .KIHCAVKSL NRITDIGEVS QFLTEGIIMK
C-ErbB GSGAFGTVYK GLWIP.EGEK VKIPVAIKEL REATSPKANK EILDEAYVMA
C-Src GQGCFGEVWM GTW......N GTTRVAIKTL KPGTMSPE.. AFLQEAQVMK
C-Kit GAGAFGKVVE ATAYGLIKSD AAMTVAVKML KPSAHLTERE ALMSELKVLS
Ret GEGEFGKVVK ATAFHLKGRA GYTTVAVKML KENASPSELR DLLSEFNVLK
Met DF.SHPNVLS LLGICLRSEG SPLVVLPYMK HGDLRNFIRN ETH.......
C-ErbB SV.DNPHVCR LLGICLTS.. TVQLITQLMP YGCLLDYIRE HKD.......
C-Src KL.RHEKLVQ LYAVV..SEE PIYIVTEYMS KGSLLDFLKG EMGKY.....
C-Kit YLGNHMNIVN LLGAC.TIGG PTLVITEYCC YGDLLNFLRR KRDSFICSKQ
Ret QV.NHPHVIK LYGAC.SQDG PLLLIVEYAK YGSLRGFLRE SR........
Met ....
C-ErbB ....
C-Src ....
C-Kit EDHAEAALYK NLLHSKESSC SDSTNEYMDM KPGVSYVVPT KADKRRSVRI
Ret .... KVGPGYLGSG GSRNSSSLD.
1206
1213
Catalytic loop
Met ....NP TVKDLIGFGL QVAKAMKYLA SKKFVHRDLA
C-ErbB ....NI GSQYLLNWCV QIAKGMNYLE ERRLVHRDLA
C-Src ....L RLPQLVDMAA QIASGMAYVE RMNYVHRDLR
C-Kit GSYIERDVTP AIMEDDELAL DLEDLLSFSY QVAKGMAFLA SKNCIHRDLA
Ret ....HPDERAL TMGDLISFAW QISQGMQYLA EMKLVHRDLA
Activation loop
1238
1246
1248
1268
Met ARNCMLDEKF TVKVADFGLA RDM..YDKEY YSVHNKTGAK LPVKWMALES
C-ErbB ARNVLVKTPQ HVKITDFGLA KLLGADEKEY HA....EGGK VPIKWMALES
C-Src AANILVGENL VCKVADFGLA RLIEDNE... ..YTARQGAK FPIKWTAPEA
C-Kit ARNILLTHGR ITKICDFGLA RDIKNDS... .NYVVKGNAR LPVKWMAPES
Ret ARNILVAEGR KMKISDFGLS RDVYEED... .SYVKRSQGR IPVKWMAIES
D816V-Mastocytosis
D820G-Mastocytosis
M918T-MEN2B

RCCs, and of PRCs in particular, and stress the importance of the classification of renal neoplasms based on combined pathological and molecular genetic criteria.

Heterogeneity of Papillary Renal Carcinoma

The association between MET mutations and a particular histologic subtype of PRC is remarkable. Previously, we emphasized that germline mutations in the VHL and MET genes predispose to specific histologic types of renal neoplasia. Mutations in the VHL tumor-suppressor gene predispose to clear cell renal carcinoma; mutations in the MET proto-oncogene predispose to PRC. This report emphasizes that mutations in MET predispose to a specific subtype of papillary renal cancer suggesting that PRC is genetically heterogeneous. This concept is reinforced by the identification of families with PRC type 2; affected members of these families do not have germline MET mutations (Zbar, Lubensky, Schmidt, Merino and Linehan, unpubl. data).

The morphologic appearance of PRCs produced by t(x;1) chromosomal translocation resulting in somatic mutations in the TFE3 and PPRC genes is different from the morphology associated with germline or somatic MET mutations [12–16] (Lubensky and Linehan, unpubl. observations).

Classification of Inherited Carcinomas of the Kidney

In order to place into perspective the association of mutations in the MET proto-oncogene with PRC type 1 (HPRC1), it is useful to consider the inherited tumors of the kidney. Virtually all inherited clear cell carcinomas of the kidney are produced by mutations in the VHL gene [8]. This group includes VHL disease families, as well as families with constitutional translocations involving chromosome 3p [17–20]. Tumorigenesis in families with constitutional chromosomal translocations is associated with loss of the derivative chromosome carrying distal 3p and somatic mutation of the remaining VHL

Fig. 1. Partial amino acid sequence of the tyrosine kinase domain of MET illustrating location of germline and somatic mutations in papillary renal carcinomas (shown in red). The amino acid sequences of the homologous regions of c-erbB, c-src, c-Kit and RET are shown for comparison; conserved codons are in blue. The locations of the RET mutations,E768D, L790F, Y791F, V804L, and M918T are shown; the locations of the mutations in c-Kit that produce mastocytosis with an associated hematologic disorder, D816V, and D820G, are indicated; the location of the V157I mutation in c-erbB that produces malignancy is shown. From Schmidt et al. [11].

gene [18, 19]. A few families with multiple members affected with clear cell renal carcinoma have been described in which the predisposing gene is not known [21]. Also, a recently recognized familial form of renal oncocytoma has been identified but the gene responsible for this inherited benign tumor of the kidney remains unidentified [22].

The inherited PRCs of the kidney may be divided into two groups. HPRC1 refers to hereditary PRCs produced by germline mutations in the MET proto-oncogene. Inherited PRCs without mutations in the MET proto-oncogene are classified as HPRC2. The gene(s) responsible for an inherited predisposition to PRC type 2 is not known.

Cytogenetic Studies of Papillary Renal Carcinomas

The karyotype of PRCs has been described by Kovacs [16] using classic cytogenetic techniques, and more recently, by fluorescent microsatellite analysis [23]. Papillary adenomas of the kidney were characterized by trisomy of chromosomes 7 and 17, and in men, by loss of the Y chromosome. Papillary carcinomas of the kidney were characterized by trisomy of chromosomes 7, 12, 16, 17, and 20.

Recently, the issue of chromosomal changes in PRCs was revisited by Jiang et al. [4] who analyzed a series of PRCs by comparative genomic hybridization. These workers found significant genetic differences between PRC types 1 and 2. Trisomy 7 and trisomy 17 were significantly less frequent in PRC type 2 compared to PRC type 1. Other chromosomal gains and losses were detected but there was no significant difference in the frequency of these changes between PRC types 1 and 2. Although Jiang et al. [4] detected gains of copies of chromosomes 12, 16 or 20 in PRCs, there was no correlation between the frequency of these chromosomal gains, and the stage or grade of the papillary neoplasm.

Clonality of Papillary Renal Carcinomas in Affected Members of HPRC Families

Patients with HPRC1 have bilateral, multiple PRCs. One important question is whether these tumors are independent clonal events, or the result of intrarenal metastasis from a single primary tumor. Zhuang et al. [24] demonstrated that multiple PRCs from 1 female HPRC1 patient had independent clonal origins using the HUMURA assay, an assay based on inactivation of one of the X chromosomes in females during embryogenesis [24].

Nonrandom Duplication of Chromosome 7 Bearing the Mutant MET Allele in Affected Members of HPRC Families

Both Zhuang et al. [24] and Fischer et al. [25] demonstrated nonrandom duplication of chromosome 7, but random duplication of chromosome 17 in tumors from patients with HPRC1 by genotyping chromosome 7 and 17 polymorphic markers and determining allele ratios by phosphoimaging analysis. Haplotyping the region immediately adjacent to the MET gene showed that the chromosome 7 bearing the mutant MET allele was the chromosome duplicated in HPRC1 tumors. These data strongly suggest that 2 copies of the mutant MET gene are required for the development of papillary renal tumors in patients with HPRC1.

Taken together, this information indicates that each papillary renal tumor in patients with HPRC1 arises as an independent clonal event. Probably, duplication of chromosome 7 occurs randomly in renal cells. Only those cells, which duplicate the chromosome 7 bearing the mutant MET allele, continue to proliferate to form a detectable renal neoplasm. Whether there are processes which favor chromosome duplication is not known.

Selection of Chromosome 7q31 and Chromosome 17q in Renal Tumors

Glukhova et al. [26] serially transplanted grafts of human PRCs in nude mice. Successful transplantation of the xenografts was associated with enrichment of cytogenetic changes present in the primary tumor [26]. The xenografts were enriched for duplication of chromosome 7q31 and chromosome 17q21-qter. It is not known whether the MET gene was mutated in the xenografts, or whether the expression of MET was increased; an increased number of copies of MET was demonstrated in some tumors. These results support the idea that the chromosomal regions 7q31 and 17q21-qter contain genes whose expression is critical to the growth and proliferation of human PRCs.

Number of Renal Tumors in Patients with HPRC

There is considerable variation in the number of PRCs in patients with the identical germline MET mutation, for example, H1112R. One patient in family 150, III-18, had at least 100 PRCs; his 2 brothers, carriers of the H1112R mutation, and of similar age, had a total of 1 renal tumor [6] (unpubl. data, Zbar and Linehan). The factors underlying this considerable variability are unknown, but may indicate a role of modifier genes that may be required for complete expression of the PRC phenotype.

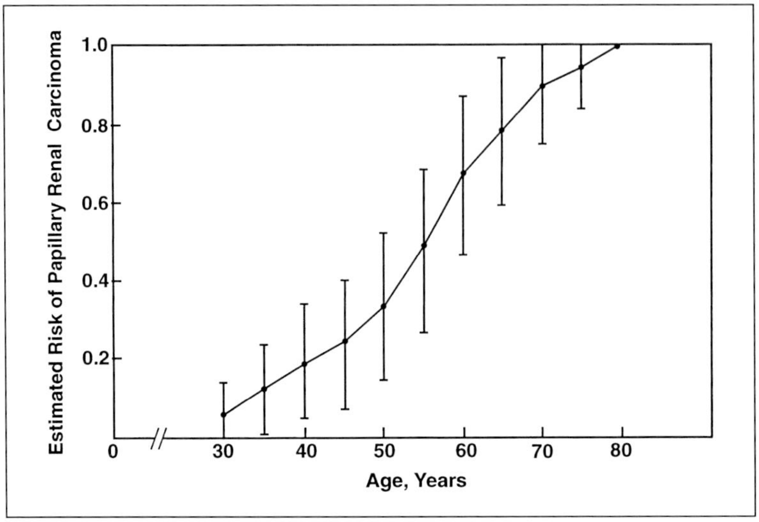

Fig. 2. Penetrance of the H1112R MET mutation. The mutation status was determined by sequencing exon 16 of the MET gene. Renal tumor status was determined by CT or by pathological examination of resected tumor samples. Kaplan-Meier plots were generated by the computer program of Thomas et al. From Schmidt et al. [10].

Age of Tumor Development

The age of development of PRCs is best studied in the context of the MET H1112R mutation. The risk estimation curve (fig. 2) plotting fraction of patients with renal neoplasms (detected by computerized tomography) as a function of patient age indicates that by age of 55, only half of the H1112R mutation carriers have developed detectable disease [10]. Although the MET mutations produce changes that can be measured in short-term assays in vitro, in humans these MET mutations require years to become manifest. This delay in tumor development may reflect the time required for duplication of the mutant MET allele, the development of trisomy of other chromosomes (chromosome 17, for example) and/or the action of proteins produced by modifier genes.

MET and Metastasis: Studies in Patients

Do patients with PRCs as a consequence of mutations in the MET proto-oncogene develop metastases? This question is best addressed in families with the MET H1112R mutation, because the number of patients with this mutation is great [10]. There are 23 individuals carrying the germline H1112R mutation who are affected with PRC; there are 15 asymptomatic carriers of the H1112R MET mutation. Of the 23 individuals known to have papillary renal tumors associated with the H1112R MET mutation, 6 (26%) had distant metastases.

Frequency of MET Mutations in Patients with Sporadic Papillary Renal Carcinoma

Schmidt et al. [11] have reported that 13% of sporadic PRCs had mutations in the MET proto-oncogene. In this work, the denominator was all PRCs studied without regard for PRC subtypes. If we assume that 50% of sporadic PRCs are type 1, and use as the denominator the number of sporadic PRC type 1 tumors, the frequency of MET mutation in sporadic PRC might be as high as 25%.

MET/HGF Receptor/Ligand Signaling System

The MET proto-oncogene encodes a transmembrane receptor tyrosine kinase protein whose ligand is hepatocyte growth factor/scatter factor (HGF/SF). The MET protein is widely expressed in epithelial cells; HGF is produced primarily by mesenchymal cells. The MET/HGF receptor/ligand pair mediates several important biological processes including cell proliferation, motility, differentiation, as well as normal embryological development [27]. These biological activities have been measured in vitro by assays of the proliferation and movement of cells [28], and by formation of tubular structures in response to receptor/ligand signaling [29]; in addition genetic engineering studies have been performed in mice [30, 31].

The critical element in MET/HGF receptor/ligand signaling is autophosphorylation. Ligand binding to the MET protein triggers receptor dimerization and phosphorylation of other MET molecules in trans. Subsequent downstream phosphorylation of a src-2 homology (SH2)-docking site located in the COOH terminal tail of the MET protein permits binding of SH2-containing second-messenger molecules and activates MET/HGF signaling pathways [32]. Molecular modeling studies suggest that the inactive form of the MET receptor is autoinhibited by the activation loop of the tyrosine kinase domain. Binding of the ligand HGF facilitates the conversion of the inactive (unphosphorylated) form of the MET receptor to the active (phosphorylated) form [33].

The 16 tyrosine residues in the intracellular domain of the MET protein (designated Y1-Y16) have been evaluated for their role in MET/HGF signaling. Binding of its ligand HGF to the extracellular domain of the MET receptor stimulates autophosphorylation on tyrosines 1252 and 1253 (Y8 and Y9) in the activation loop of the tyrosine kinase. (Numbering is in accordance with Genbank Accession No. J02958.) This phosphorylation event is critical to all subsequent steps. Mutation of Y1252 and Y1253 to phenylalanines blocked all HGF-induced signaling [33].

Signal transduction by HGF/MET requires phosphorylation of tyrosines 1367 and 1374 (Y14 and Y15) located in the COOH terminal tail of the protein. Upon phosphorylation, this region interacts with many SH2 domain-containing signal transducer proteins. The SH2 domains of phosphoinositol 3-kinase (PI 3-K), phospholipase, C gamma 1 (PLC γ), and pp60 c-src bind directly to either of the phosphotyrosines in consensus sequence Y1367 VHVNAT-Y1374 VNV, the 11 amino acid multifunctional docking site. Grb2/SOS (growth factor receptor binding protein 2/son-of-sevenless complex) binds specifically to the motif, Y1374VNV, and acts as an adaptor for Gab-1, a multiadaptor protein. Gab-1 coupling to the MET/Grb2 complex facilitates the binding of PLC γ and the p85 subunit of PI 3-K to MET in a Grb 2-dependent manner [32].

The critical role of tyrosines 1367 and 1374 in the SH2-docking site has been established with mouse model studies. Homozygous mice carrying a Y1367, Y1374→F1367, F1374 mutated MET died in utero in the same time frame as MET knockout mice [31], proving the essential role of the multifunctional docking site for mouse development. The YY→FF mutation in oncogenic TPR-MET abrogated transformation and experimental metastasis, underscoring the role of MET signaling in cell proliferation, invasion and metastasis [34].

Blocking the ability of MET to signal through the Ras pathway by transfecting MDCK cells with dominant-negative Ras led to inhibition of cell motility [28]. Mutation of the Grb2 consensus sequence, N1376→H1376, blocked cellular transformation initiated by TPR-MET [35], and in mouse studies led to impaired limb development but not liver or placenta [31], supporting the role of the Ras pathway in cell motility and transformation. Duplication of the Grb2 site enhanced in vitro transformation but abolished metastatic potential, indicating the requirement of other signal transducers for invasion and metastases [35].

Recent studies [36] suggest a role for Y6 and Y10 in MET/HGF signaling. Substitution of these tyrosines for phenylalanines in a wild-type MET construct, coexpressing HGF in NIH3T3 cells, significantly diminished this oncogenic MET/HGF autocrine signaling.

MET/HGF Receptor/Ligand Pair in Cancer

The MET/HGF receptor ligand pair has been implicated in the pathogenesis of human cancer. MET overexpression has been documented in a large number of malignancies including thyroid carcinoma, pancreatic carcinoma, osteosarcomas, glioblastomas, and colon cancer [37]. The biochemical basis for the overexpression of MET protein in human cancers is not understood. There is no evidence for genomic amplification of the MET gene in most cancers with overexpression of the protein; however, there has been some suggestion of increased transcription of the MET message.

The recent identification of germline and somatic mutations in the tyrosine kinase domain of MET in patients with PRC established a direct link between the MET receptor tyrosine kinase and human cancer. Germline MET mutations were identified in affected members of 6 of 7 families with HPRC [9, 10]. The mutations were shown to segregate with disease phenotype. In addition, mutations were identified in 13% of sporadic PRCs from patients with no family history of renal cancer [11]. All mutations were missense and were located in the tyrosine kinase domain of the MET proto-oncogene. It is interesting that three PRC-associated MET mutations are located in 'hot spots', codons homologous to codons where disease-causing mutations have been found in RET, c-Kit and c-erbB, other receptor tyrosine kinases (fig. 1). To date 15 different mutations have been identified in 10 codons (table 1).

The identification of MET mutations in PRC has raised a number of questions. How do these missense mutations in MET lead to cancer? Are these missense mutations in MET gain-of-function mutations? How do these mutant MET molecules signal? What biological processes are altered by mutations in MET? How can mutant MET activities be inhibited? How can one visualize the 3D structure of the mutant MET receptor? Are dimers formed by mutant MET?

Activating Mutations in MET Vary in Transforming Ability

Studies by Jeffers et al. [38] showed that the missense mutations in the tyrosine kinase domain of MET associated with PRC stimulate transformation when transfected into NIH3T3 cells as measured by focus formation. Strong activating mutations (i.e. M1268T) produced >300 transformed foci per microgram of DNA, intermediate activating mutations (i.e. Y1248H, D1246N, D1246H, Y1248C) produced 100–200 transformed foci, and no transformed foci were produced by the weak activating mutants (i.e. M1149T, V1238I, V1206L). Mutations which originated from sporadic PRC were generally more activating than those carried in the germline.

Mutations in MET are Gain-of-Function Mutations

When biochemical studies were performed on NIH 3T3 cells expressing exogenous wild-type or mutant MET protein, several observations were consistently made. Although the amount of exogenous MET protein made by NIH 3T3 cells expressing wild-type or mutant MET molecules was similar, there were major differences in MET phosphorylation on tyrosine, and kinase activity between cells transfected with wild-type MET and mutant MET genes. Cells expressing mutant MET showed increased MET kinase activity compared to cells expressing wild-type MET; mutant MET proteins were phosphorylated on tyrosine in the absence of the ligand, HGF; wild-type MET proteins did not show ligand-independent phosphorylation [38].

Biological Processes Altered by Activating MET Mutations

Cells expressing exogenous activating mutant MET proteins exhibit a number of characteristics not found in cells expressing exogenous wild-type MET. These characteristics include the formation of foci in monolayers of transfected NIH 3T3 cells, the scattering of Madin Darby canine kidney cells, and the formation of tumors in immunodeficient mice inoculated with mutant MET transfected NIH 3T3 cells [38, 39]. In addition, NIH 3T3 cells expressing exogenous mutant MET or NIH 3T3 cells expressing exogenous Trk-mutant MET chimeric protein form pulmonary metastases when injected intravenously into immunodeficient mice [39].

Signaling Pathways Used by Activating Mutant MET Molecules

NIH 3T3 cells transfected with activating mutant MET molecules appear to signal through the same pathways used by wild-type MET molecules. In NIH 3T3 cells transfected with MET mutants Y1248H, D1246H, D1246N and M1268T, mutant MET molecules were constitutively associated with Gab1, Grb2/SOS and the p85 subunit of PI 3-K suggesting that mutant MET binds to the same signal transducers as wild-type MET. Mutation of the 2 tyrosines in the SH2-docking site completely abrogated the association of mutant MET molecules with downstream signal transducers and inhibited transformation of NIH 3T3 cells [40].

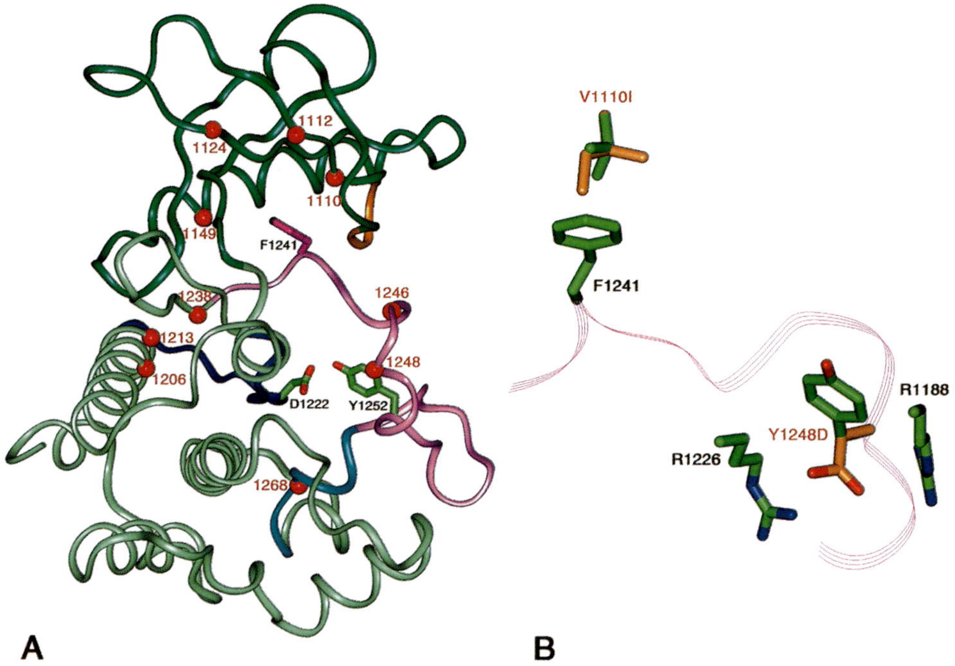

Fig. 3. 3D model of the kinase domain of MET in the autoinhibited form. *A* Ribbon representation of the protein backbone. N-terminal and C-terminal lobes are shown in dark and light green, respectively; the glycine-rich, ATP-binding loop in orange, the catalytic loop in dark blue, the activation loop in magenta, the P+1 loop in blue. The position of MET-activating mutations are marked as red dots. *B* Selected side chains of wild-type (green) and mutated (orange) MET residues. The replacement of valine 1110 with isoleucine results in a steric clash with phenylalanine 1241. Substitution of tyrosine 1248 with aspartic acid eliminates the hydrophobic interactions of the phenolic ring of Y1248 with the aliphatic side chains of arginines 1226 and 1188 which stabilize the inhibitory conformation of the activation loop. Both mutations will facilitate the transition to the active form of the enzyme. From Schmidt et al. [11].

Knowledge Gained by Molecular Modeling of MET Mutant Molecules

Molecular modeling of the MET tyrosine kinase domain on the insulin receptor kinase crystal structure suggests that in the inactive (unphosphorylated) state, the kinase activity of the protein is inhibited by placement of the COOH terminal tail of the protein into the active site of the molecule (fig. 3) [11]. The COOH terminal tail of the MET protein acts as a pseudosubstrate and both the ATP and substrate-binding domains of the MET kinase are inaccesible to cytosol. The mutations identified in PRC patients appear to destabilize the inactive conformation of the MET molecule facilitating transition to the active state. Visualized as a light switch, in cells containing mutant MET receptors the switch is not in the 'off' position; the switch is located between the 'off' and 'on' positions. This interpretation is reinforced by the finding that when the ligand HGF is added to cells expressing exogenous mutant MET molecules, the number of foci formed by NIH 3T3 cells is greater than the number of foci formed when cells expressing exogenous wild-type MET are treated with HGF. The mutations in MET increase the responsiveness of cells to the ligand HGF [39].

MET and Metastasis: Studies in Experimental Animals

Recent experimental studies by Jeffers et al. [39] and Bardelli et al. [40] implicated the MET proto-oncogene in the metastatic process. When NIH 3T3 cells transfected with mutant MET genes were injected intravenously into athymic nude mice, tumor deposits formed in the lungs. Pulmonary metastases also formed after injection of NIH 3T3 cells transfected with the extracellular ligand-binding domain of nerve growth factor fused to the intracellular mutant MET tyrosine kinase domain. Mice bearing a mutant MET transgene under the control of the metallothionien promoter formed breast cancers with metastases.

Conclusions

Activating mutations in the tyrosine kinase domain of the MET receptor lead to a predisposition to develop bilateral, multiple PRCs. These PRCs are of a specific histologic subtype, PRC type 1. Systemic metastases occurred in a subset of patients with the H1112R germline mutation.

Activating mutations, to date, have been identified only in the tyrosine kinase domain of the MET protein. The location of three mutations in MET correspond to 'hot spots', that is, to codons located in other receptor tyrosine kinases that when mutated produce receptor activation, and disease. Signaling studies indicate that NIH 3T3 cells expressing activating MET mutations show constitutive phosphorylation of the MET tyrosine kinase, increased kinase activity, and constitutive binding of signaling effectors, Gab1, Grb2/SOS, and the p85 subunit of PI 3-K. Signaling of activating mutant MET receptors proceeds through at least some of the same pathways used by ligand-stimulated, wild-type MET molecules.

Acknowledgments

The content of this publication does not necessarily reflect the views or policies of the Department of Health and Human Services, nor does mention of trade names, commercial products, or organizations imply endorsement by the US Government. This project has been funded in part with Federal funds from the National Cancer Institute, National Institutes of Health, under Contract No. NO1-CO-56000.

References

1 Thoenes W, Storkel S, Rumpelt HJ: Histopathology and classification of renal tumors (adenomas, oncocytomas and carcinomas). The basic cytological and histopathological elements and their use for diagnostics. Pathol Res Pract 1986;181:125–143.
2 Kovacs G: Papillary renal cell carcinoma. A morphologic and cytogenetic study of 11 cases. Am J Pathol 1989;134:27–34.
3 Delahunt B, Eble JN: Papillary renal cell carcinoma: A clinicopathologic and immunohistochemical study of 105 tumors. Mod Pathol 1997;10:537–544.
4 Jiang F, Richter J, Schraml P, Bubendorf L, Gasser T, Sauter G, Mihatsch MJ, Moch H: Chromosomal imbalances in papillary renal cell carcinoma: Genetic differences between histological subtypes. Am J Pathol 1998;153:1467–1473.
5 Amin MB, Corless CL, Renshaw AA, Tickoo SK, Kubus J, Schultz DS: Papillary (chromophil) renal cell carcinoma: Histomorphological characteristics and evaluation of conventional pathologic prognostic parameters in 62 cases. Am J Surg Pathol 1997;21:621–635.
6 Zbar B, Tory K, Merino M, Schmidt L, Glenn G, Choyke P, Walther MM, Lerman M, Linehan WM: Hereditary papillary renal cell carcinoma. J Urol 1994;151:561–566.
7 Zbar B, Glenn G, Lubensky I, Choyke P, Walther MM, Magnusson G, Bergerheim USR, Pettersson S, Amin M, Hurley K, Linehan WM: Hereditary papillary renal cell carcinoma: Clinical studies in 10 families. J Urol 1995;153:907–912.
8 Zbar B, Lerman M: Inherited carcinomas of the kidney. Adv Cancer Res 1998;75:163–201.
9 Schmidt L, Duh F-M, Chen F, Kishida T, Glenn G, Choyke P, Scherer S, Zhuang Z, Lubensky I, Dean M, Allikmets R, Chidambaram A, Bergerheim UR, Feltis JT, Casadevall C, Zamarron A, Bernues M, Richard S, Lips CJM, Walther MM, Tsui L-C, Geil L, Orcutt ML, Stackhouse T, Lipan J, Slife L, Brauch H, Decker J, Niehans G, Hughson MD, Moch H, Storkel S, Lerman MI, Linehan WM, Zbar B: Germline and somatic mutations in the tyrosine kinase domain of the MET proto-oncogene in papillary renal carcinomas. Nat Genet 1997;16:68–73.
10 Schmidt L, Junker K, Weirich G, Glenn G, Choyke P, Lubensky I, Zhuang Z, Jeffers M, Vande Woude G, Neumann H, Walther M, Linehan, WM, Zbar B: Two North American families with hereditary papillary renal carcinoma and identical novel mutations in the MET proto-oncogene. Cancer Res 1998;58:1719–1722.
11 Schmidt L, Junker K, Nakaigawa N, Kinjerski T, Weirich G, Miller M, Lubensky I, Neumann HPH, Brauch H, Decker J, Vocke C, Brown JA, Jenkins R, Richard S, Bergerheim U, Gerrard B, Dean M, Linehan WM, Zbar B: Novel mutations in the MET proto-oncogene in papillary renal carcinomas. Oncogene 1999;18:2343–2350.
12 Weterman MAJ, Wilbrink M, Geurts van Kessel A: Fusion of the transcription factor TFE3 gene to a novel gene, PRCC, in t(X;1)(p11;q21)-positive papillary renal cell carcinomas. Proc Natl Acad Sci USA 1996;93:15294–15298.
13 Weterman MA, Wilbrink M, Janssen I, Janssen HA, van den Berg E, Fisher SE, Craig I, Geurts Van Kessel A: Molecular cloning of the papillary renal cell carcinoma-associated translocation (X; 1)(p11;q21) breakpoint. Cytogenet Cell Genet 1996;75:2–6.
14 Clark J, Lu YJ, Sidhar SK, Parker C, Gill S, Smedley D, Hamoudi R, Linehan WM, Shipley J, Cooper CS: Fusion of splicing factor genes PSF and NonO (p54nrb) to the TFE3 gene in papillary renal cell carcinoma. Oncogene 1997;15:2233–2239.

15 Sidhar SK, Clark J, Gill S, Hamoudi R, Crew AJ, Gwilliam R, Ross M, Linehan WM, Birdsall S, Shipley J, Cooper CS: The t(X;1) (p11.2;q21.2) translocation in papillary renal cell carcinoma fuses a novel gene PRCC to the TFE3 transcription factor gene. Hum Mol Genet 1996;5:1333–1338.
16 Kovacs G. Molecular cytogenetics of renal cell tumors. Adv Cancer Res 1993;62:89–124.
17 Li FP, Decker H-J H, Zbar B, Stanton VP, Kovacs G, Seizinger B, Aburantani H, Sandberg AA, Berg S, Hosoe S, Brown R: Clinical and genetic studies of renal cell carcinomas in a family with a constitutional chromosome 3:8 translocation. Ann Intern Med 1993;118:106–111.
18 Schmidt L, Li F, Brown RS, Berg S, Chen F, Wei M-W, Tory K, Lerman MI, Zbar B: Mechanism of tumorigenesis of renal carcinomas associated with the constitutional chromosome 3;8 translocation. Cancer J Sci Am 1995;1:191–196.
19 Bodmer D, Eleveld MJ, Ligtenberg MJ, Weterman MA, Janssen BA, Smeets DF, de Wit PE, van den Berg A, van den Berg E, Koolen MI, Geurts van Kessel A: An alternative route for multistep tumorigenesis in a novel case of hereditary renal cell cancer and a t(2;3)(q35;q21) chromosome translocation. Am J Hum Genet 1998;62:1475–1483.
20 van den Berg A, van der Veen AY, Hulsbeek MM, Kovacs G, Gemmill RM, Drabkin HA, Buys CH: Defining the position of the breakpoint of the constitutional t(3;6) occurring in a family with renal cell carcinoma. Genes Chromosomes Cancer 1995;12:224–228.
21 Teh BT, Giraud S, Sari NF, Hii SI, Bergerat JP, Larsson C, Limarcher JM, Nicol D: Familial non-VHL non papillary clear-cell renal cancer. Lancet 1997;349:848–849.
22 Weirich G, Glenn G, Junker K, Merino M, Storkel S, Lubensky I, Choyke P, Pack S, Amin M, Walther MM, Linehan WM, Zbar B: Familial renal oncocytoma: Clinicopathological study of 5 families. J Urol 1998;160:335–340.
23 Bugert P, Kovacs G: Molecular differential diagnosis of renal cell carcinomas by microsatellite analysis. Am J Pathol 1996;149:2081–2088.
24 Zhuang Z, Park WS, Pack S, Schmidt L, Vortmeyer AO, Pak E, Pham T, Weil RJ, Candidus S, Lubensky IA, Linehan WM, Zbar B, Weirich G: Trisomy 7-harbouring non-random duplication of the mutant MET allele in hereditary papillary renal carcinomas. Nat Genet 1998;20:66–69.
25 Fischer J, Palmedo G, von Knobloch R, Bugert P, Prayer-Galetti T, Pagano F, Kovacs G: Duplication and overexpression of the mutant allele of the MET proto-oncogene in multiple hereditary papillary renal cell tumors. Oncogene 1998;17:733–739.
26 Glukhova L, Goguel AF, Chuboda I, Angevin E, Pavon C, Terrier-Lacombe MJ, Meddeb M, Escudier B, Bernheim A: Overrepresentation of 7q31 and 17q in renal cell carcinomas. Genes Chromosomes Cancer 1998;22:171–178.
27 Comoglio PM, Vigna E: Structure and functions of the HGF receptor (c-Met); in Jirtle R (ed): Liver Regeneration and Carcinogenesis. New York, Academic Press, 1995, pp 51–70.
28 Hartmann G, Weidner KM, Schwartz H, Birchmeier W: The motility signal of scatter factor/hepatocyte growth factor mediated through the receptor tyrosine kinase Met requires intracellular action of Ras. J Biol Chem 1994;269:21936–21939.
29 Santos O, Barros E, Yang X, Matsumoto K, Nakamura T, Park M, Nigam S: Involvement of hepatocyte growth factor in kidney development. Dev Biol 1994;163:525–529.
30 Schmidt C, Bladt F, Goedecke S, Brinkmann V, Zschiesche W, Sharpe M, Gherardi E, Birchmeier C: Scatter factor/hepatocyte growth factor is essential for liver development. Nature 1995;373:699–702.
31 Maina F, Casagranda F, Audero E, Simeone A, Comoglio P, Klein RA, Ponzetto C: Uncoupling of Grb2 from the Met receptor in vivo reveals complex roles in muscle development. Cell 1996;87:531–542.
32 Bardelli A, Pugliese L, Comoglio PM: 'Invasive-growth' signaling by the Met/HGF receptor. The hereditary renal carcinoma connection. Biochem Biophys Acta 1997;1333:M41-M51.
33 Longati P, Bardelli A, Ponzetto C, Naldini L, Comoglio PM: Tyrosines 1234–1235 are critical for activation of the tyrosine kinase encoded by the MET proto-oncogene (HGF receptor). Oncogene 1994;9:49–57.
34 Ponzetto C, Bardelli A, Zhen Z, Maina F, dalla Zonca P, Giordano S, Graziani A, Panayotou G, Comoglio P: A multifunctional docking site mediates signaling and transformation by the hepatocyte growth factor/scatter factor receptor family. Cell 1994;77:261–271.

35 Ponzetto C, Zhen Z, Audero E, Mania F, Bardelli A, Basile ML, Giordano S, Narsimhan R, Comoglio P: Specific uncoupling of Grb2 from the Met receptor. Cell 1996;271:14119–14123.
36 Jeffers M, Koochekpour S, Fiscella M, Sathyanarayana BK, Vande Woude GF: Signaling requirements for oncogenic forms of the MET tyrosine kinase receptor. Oncogene 1998;17:2691–2700.
37 Jeffers M, Rong S, vande Woude G: Hepatocyte growth factor/scatter factor-MET signaling in tumorigenicity and invasion/metastasis. J Mol Med 1996;74:505–513.
38 Jeffers M, Schmidt L, Nakaigawa N, Webb CP, Weirich G, Kishida T, Zbar B, Vande Woude G: Activating mutations for the MET tyrosine kinase receptor in human cancer. Proc Natl Acad Sci USA 1997;94:11445–11450.
39 Jeffers M, Fiscella M, Webb CP, Anver M, Koochekpour S, Vande Woude GF: The mutationally activated MET receptor mediates motility and metastasis. Proc Natl Acad Sci USA 1998;95:14417–14422.
40 Bardelli A, Longati P, Gramaglia D, Basilico C, Tamagnone L, Giordano S, Ballinari D, Michieli P, Comoglio PM: Uncoupling signal transducers from oncogenic MET mutants abrogates cell transformation and inhibits invasive growth. Proc Natl Acad Sci USA 1998;95:14379–14383.

Dr. Laura Schmidt, Intramural Research Support Program, SAIC Frederick,
Building 560, Room 12-34, National Cancer Institute-Frederick Cancer Research and
Development Center, Frederick, MD 21702 (USA)
Tel. +1 301 846 1288, Fax +1 301 846 6145, E-Mail schmidtl@mail.ncifcrf.gov

Hino O (ed): Kidney Cancer. Recent Results of Basic and Clinical Research.
Contrib Nephrol. Basel, Karger, 1999, vol 128, pp 28–44

Renal Cell Carcinomas in Patients on Long-Term Hemodialysis

Isao Ishikawa

Division of Nephrology, Department of Internal Medicine, Kanazawa Medical University, Uchinada, Japan

Introduction

Renal cell carcinoma (RCC) is an important complication of long-term hemodialysis. At present (December 1998), over 700,000 patients worldwide (280,000 in the United States, 176,000 in Japan and 160,000 in Europe) are being treated for end-stage renal diseases by either hemodialysis or continuous ambulatory peritoneal dialysis (CAPD). The number of patients is growing rapidly, and many long-term dialysis patients undergo dialysis for more than 10 years. For example, 40,000 patients or 23% of all dialysis patients are long-term dialysis patients in Japan [1] because few renal transplantations are performed. Acquired renal cystic disease with or without RCC [2–5] is one of the new diseases that develops in patients on long-term dialysis due to conditions such as dialysis amyloidosis, aluminum intoxication and accelerated atherosclerosis. In 1977, Dunnill et al. [2] described acquired cystic disease of the kidney in 14 of 30 autopsy cases, 6 of which exhibited a renal tumor, including 1 metastasis. In this study RCC in dialysis patients is reviewed.

Our First Case

In 1978, we encountered the first patient who successfully underwent surgery for RCC. The subject was a 24-year-old male who had been treated by hemodialysis for 7 years [3]. The diagnostic process in this case was unusual. His preoperative and initial postoperative diagnoses were infected autosomal dominant polycystic kidney disease and autosomal dominant polycystic kidney disease with a large hematoma 7 cm in diameter, respectively. However, a renal biopsy had been performed previously which revealed crescentic glomerulonephritis.

Table 1. Gender distribution of dialysis patients with renal cell carcinoma

	1982	1984	1986	1988	1990	1992	1994	1996	1998	Total
Males	25	31	40	91	112	150	216	222	285	1,172 (80.8%)
Females	9	6	8	24	18	34	57	55	68	279 (19.2%)
Total	34	37	48	115	130	184	273	277	353	1,451

There were marked discrepancies between the findings of the surgically resected specimen and his medical history. The medical literature was reviewed at that time, and it was found that Dunnill et al. [2] had reported similar cases 1 year before. It was proposed that hemodialysis was initiated due to rapidly progressive glomerulonephritis, acquired renal cystic disease had developed during hemodialysis over a 7-year period and finally RCC developed. The pathologist was asked to reexamine the resected specimen and to focus on the hematoma. RCC of a mixed cell subtype with papillary structure was found at the wall of the hematoma. The patient exhibited acquired renal cystic disease complicated by RCC after 7 years of hemodialysis. Twenty years after nephrectomy, the patient is still on hemodialysis and is doing well, except that bladder cancer was detected 2 years prior to this study and was treated successfully.

RCC in Dialysis Patients

The prevalence of RCC in dialysis patients is 1.5% and the incidence is 0.4%/year [6]. The frequency or incidence of RCC in dialysis patients is 140 times higher than that in the general population according to our 10-year follow-up results and 3 per million per year in the general population in Japan [7, 8]. The frequency or incidence of RCC in dialysis patients is 40 times higher than that in the general population due to health examinations by sonography [8]. More precisely, the incidence is 15 times higher in males and 12 times higher in females than in the general population in Japan [9]. The last incidence data [9] showed that in patients less than 45 years of age, the incidence of RCC is 200–600 times higher than that of the general population. Gardner and Evan [10], MacDougall et al. [11] and Levine [12] reported a similar prevalence or incidence. The annual incidence of RCC is 163 of 100,000 hemodialysis patients. However, if we divide the patients according to dialysis duration, the annual incidence of RCC is 99 of 100,000 hemodialysis patients after less than 10 years, and 384 of 100,000 hemodialysis patients after more than 10 years [9].

Nationwide questionnaire studies were performed in Japan in 1982 and 1998. The total number of RCC cases was 1,451 (table 1; unpubl. data), 80.8% of which were males and 19.2% females. The male to female ratio was 4.2 to

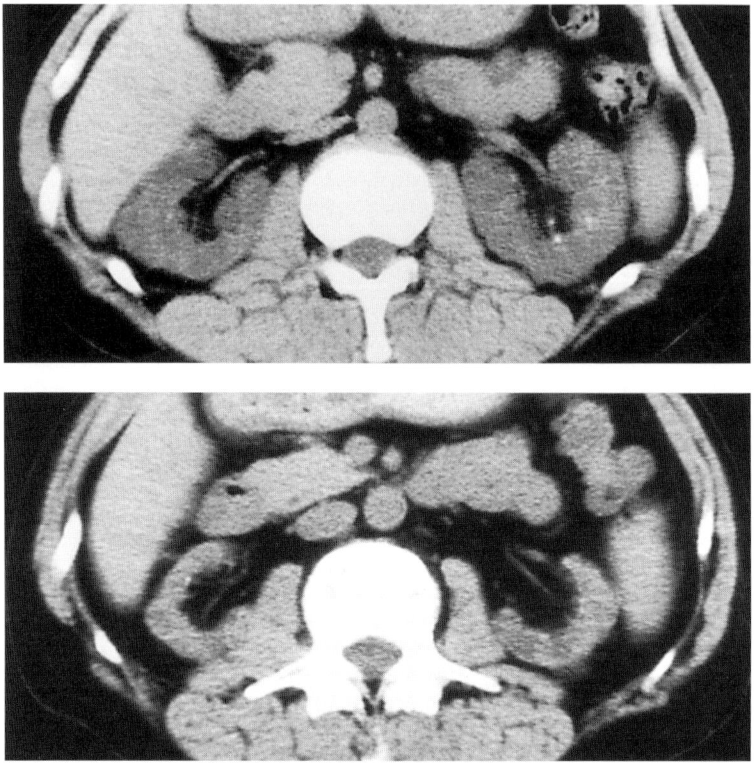

a

b

Fig. 1. Regression of acquired renal cystic disease after successful renal transplantation: *a* Acquired renal cystic disease is reflected by very low density and normal-sized kidneys in a 40-year-old male on hemodialysis for 18 years due to chronic glomerulonephritis (bilateral kidney volume 301 ml). *b* Regression of acquired cysts 3 months after transplantation (bilateral kidney volume 114 ml).

1. The mean age was 53.5 ± 11.6 years. The mean duration of hemodialysis was 115.1 ± 74.6 months. An important finding is that half of the RCC cases were found in long-term dialysis patients who had undergone dialysis for more than 10 years. The presence of acquired renal cystic disease was noted in 81.8%. Tumor size was 4.2 ± 2.9 cm. Metastasis was observed in 16% (226 of 1,411 patients) for a mean observation period of 1 year. The frequency of screening for RCC in dialysis patients was high, and RCCs in dialysis patients were cyst-related and found in long-term dialysis patients [9].

Although almost all reported cases of RCC in dialysis patients were adults, acquired renal cystic disease complicated by RCC was reported in children on dialysis [13, 14]. Therefore, age may not be relevant in the development of RCC related to cysts, and age was clearly not associated with acquired cyst development [3].

Acquired Renal Cystic Disease

Eighty percent of RCCs in dialysis patients are cyst-related RCCs. Acquired renal cystic disease is defined by bilateral development of multiple renal cysts in uremic patients with initial cyst-unrelated renal disease. The incidence and severity of acquired renal cystic disease increase in long-term dialysis patients. Acquired renal cystic disease has a male predominance [15], but is not related to age [3], dialysis modality (hemodialysis or peritoneal dialysis) [16], or dialysis membrane (cuprophan or synthetic membrane). The frequency of acquired renal cystic disease is 12, 44, 79 and 90% in patients before, <3, >3, and >10 years of hemodialysis, respectively. Marked evidence includes the regression of acquired renal cystic disease after successful renal transplantation [17] (fig. 1). Two major complications of acquired renal cystic disease are the development of a renal tumor or RCC and retroperitoneal bleeding [6, 18]. These characteristics of acquired renal cystic disease are important to understand RCC in dialysis patients.

The pathology of acquired renal cystic disease [2] suggests that a sequence of events exists in the order of tubular epithelia to cyst lining cells, hyperplastic epithelia, adenoma and finally RCC. All pathological findings for epithelial cells suggest that they are mainly derived from proximal tubules and that the risk factors for patients with developing acquired cysts and developing RCC are the same [6]. Kidneys enlarged due to acquired cysts are more likely to develop RCC [6, 19]. These indirect findings suggest a multi-step sequence from cysts to atypical cysts to adenoma to RCC [18].

RCC in CAPD Patients

The modality of treatment does not influence the development of acquired cysts or RCC [16]. No long-term CAPD patients had been reported before 1992, but 10 cases of RCC in CAPD patients were reviewed [20] and since then, more than 10 cases of RCC have been reported. Bilateral RCCs in CAPD were described recently [21].

RCC in Transplant Recipients

While acquired renal cystic disease regresses rapidly, it is assumed that the risk of RCC related to acquired renal cystic disease decreases after successful renal transplantation [17] (fig. 2). A previous study [22] reported that the incidence was 1 of 178 patients/year in dialysis patients and 1 of

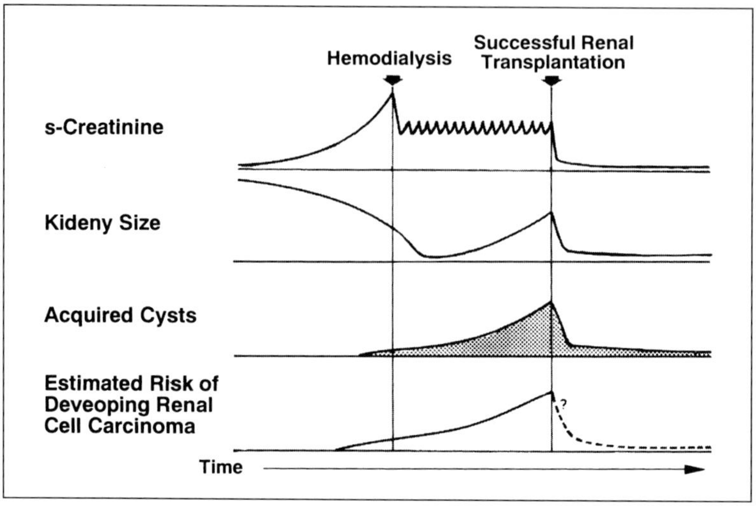

Fig. 2. Changes in serum creatinine, kidney size, severity of acquired cysts and estimated risk of developing renal cell carcinoma are illustrated during predialysis, during hemodialysis and after renal transplantation. From Ishikawa [4].

541 patients/year in transplant recipients, which supports our findings. However, this favorable condition to reduce the incidence of RCC after renal transplantation may be overcome using immunosuppressive drugs (fig. 2). In a review in 1992 [23], although the frequency of RCC in transplantation was less than that in dialysis patients, the metastatic rate of RCC found after renal transplantation was higher than that in dialysis patients. Recently, Doublet et al. [24] found RCCs in 5 of 129 recipients (3.9%) and Kliem et al. [25] reported RCCs in 12 of 154 (7.8%) patients. Sant and Ucci [26] found RCC and acquired renal cystic disease in 4 kidneys of 2 recipients. Of 19 hemodialysis patients with RCCs 92% showed no metastases, and of 7 renal transplant recipients with RCCs 71% had advanced cancer or metastasis and 3 patients died of cancer [27].

Imanishi et al. [28] reported the results of a nationwide questionnaire study of malignancy in renal transplant recipients in Japan. Of 9,010 recipients, they found 204 malignant cases, and 30 of these malignancy cases had RCCs. RCC was reported to be the most frequent type of malignancy among renal transplant recipients in Japan. Two types of RCC are diagnosed after renal transplantation: RCC which develops during the dialysis period and is diagnosed after transplantation, and RCC that develops de novo after renal transplantation. A total of 129 cases of RCC following renal transplantation was reported in 1992 [23], and more than 120 cases have been described

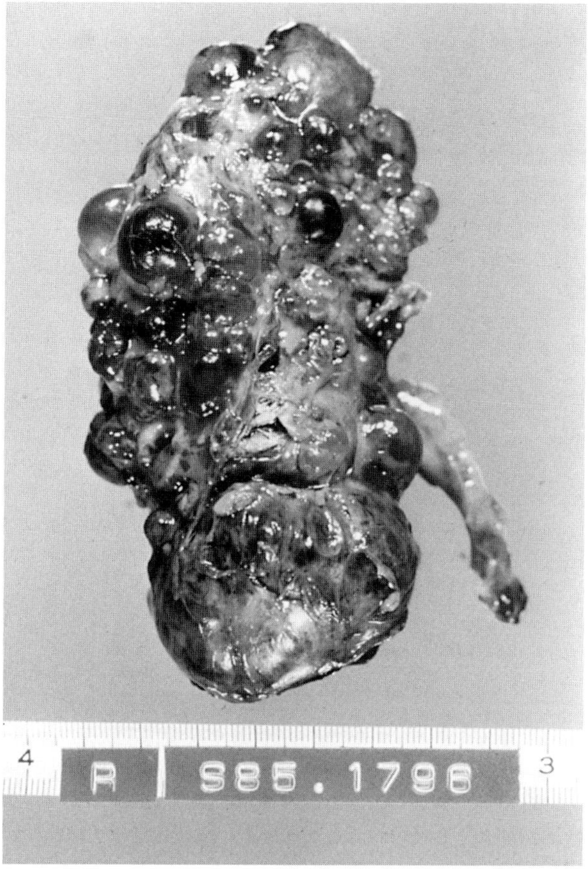

Fig. 3. Acquired renal cystic disease complicated by renal cell carcinoma. 4-cm renal cell carcinoma in the lower pole and multiple small cysts up to 2 cm are seen.

since then. The prognosis of RCC diagnosed after renal transplantation was not poor if an early diagnosis was made. Nationwide questionnaire results in Japan [28] suggest a better prognosis of RCC in transplant recipients with early detection than that previously considered. Oncocytoma in the native kidney after renal transplantation [29] has also been reported.

Histology of Acquired Renal Cystic Disease and RCC

Figure 3 illustrates acquired renal cystic disease with RCC in a long-term dialysis patient. Multiple small acquired renal cysts and RCC in the lower

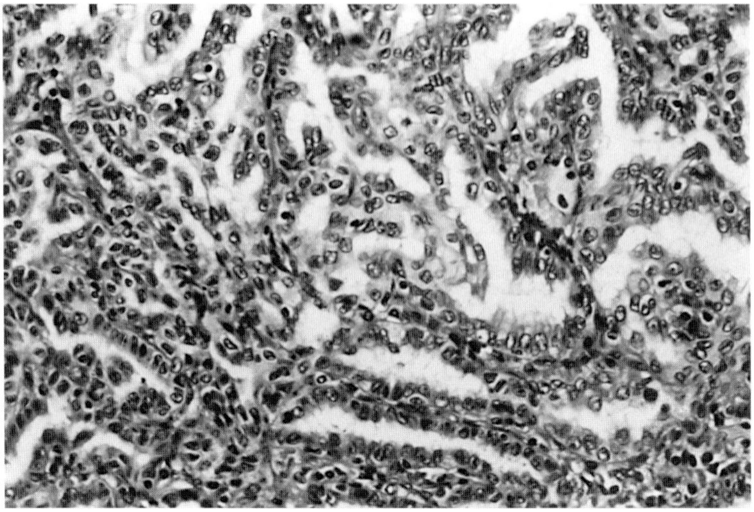

Fig. 4. Papillary renal cell carcinoma consisting of small- to medium-sized granular cells from a kidney of a 55-year-old male on hemodialysis for 140 months. ×250.

pole of the right kidney were observed. Histologically, in the majority of patients, cysts, hyperplastic epithelial cells, atypical cysts and adenomas were seen with RCC in the kidney. Tubular cells have high proliferative activity [30–33]. C-erb B2 was overexpressed in cysts, noncystic renal tissue and RCC [34]. Expression of heat shock protein was correlated with that of proliferating cell nuclear antigen [35]. The RCC and renal tumor were commonly multifocal. Therefore, a high incidence of bilateral RCC was noted in 11 of 130 cases (8.5%) [36].

Papillary and nonpapillary renal cell tumors according to Thoenes' classification in the general population can be differentiated according to their genetic constitution. The incidence of RCC in dialysis patients has been investigated histologically [37]. Nonpapillary RCC was observed in 22 cases (51.2%), whereas papillary renal cell tumors were diagnosed in 21 (48.8%) of the 43 patients treated with hemodialysis. The incidence of papillary renal cell tumors in dialysis patients is significantly higher than in the general population (4.8%). Patients with papillary renal cell tumors had received hemodialysis for a longer period than patients with nonpapillary RCCs. These data suggest that not only different genetic events but also different etiological factors are involved in the development of the two types of tumors in dialysis patients [37]. Some patients show both papillary and nonpapillary RCCs in 1 kidney [37].

The cellular and structural subtypes classified according to the 'General Rules for Clinical and Pathology Studies on Renal Cell Carcinoma supported by the Japanese Urological Association, the Japanese Society of Pathology and the Japan Radiological Society' were compared between patients on dialysis and the general population. Figure 4 reveals the granular cell subtype and papillary structure in a young, long-term dialysis patients. In 1994 and 1996, 412 RCCs in patients on dialysis were surveyed by questionnaire for cellular subtypes, and in 1996, 179 for structural subtypes. The cellular subtype was a clear subtype in 55%, granular subtype in 21% and mixed subtype in 24% of patients. Mixed and granular subtypes were significantly more predominant in patients on dialysis than in the general population, and more frequent than the clear cell subtype in patients on dialysis for more than 5 years. The structural type of RCC in patients on dialysis was alveolar in 37%, tubular in 16%, papillary in 27%, cystic in 11% and solid in 8% of the patients. Tubular and papillary types were significantly more prevalent in patients on dialysis than in the general population, and in patients on dialysis for more than 5 years. In conclusion, the cellular and structural types of RCC in patients on dialysis were slightly different from that in the general population. Granular or mixed subtype RCC with a tubular or papillary pattern is predominant in patients on long-term dialysis [9]. The hypothesis of Ishikawa and Shinoda [38] states that there are two types of RCC in dialysis patients: one occurs in older patients on short-term dialysis and is less related to acquired cysts, similar to RCC in the general population, and the other occurs at a younger age with long-term dialysis and is highly related to acquired cyst formation. The former type may show the clear cell subtype and alveolar patterns and the latter type granular or mixed cell subtypes and tubular or papillary patterns.

Besides papillary and nonpapillary RCCs, oncocytoma [39], sarcomatoid RCC [40] and Bellini's duct tumor [41] were described. Moreover, urothelial neoplasia with acquired renal cystic disease was reported [42].

Gene and Chromosomal Abnormalities in RCC in Dialysis Patients

We investigated whether there is any difference in cytogenetic abnormalities in papillary and nonpapillary RCC between dialysis patients and the general population. Trisomy 5, 16 and 20 and loss of the Y chromosome of papillary RCC were reported in a patient on long-term dialysis in 1993 [43]. We also performed karyotypic analysis in 4 papillary and 1 nonpapillary RCC cases (fig. 5) [44] and examined the loss of heterozygosity (LOH) in 4 nonpapillary RCC cases. All 4 patients with papillary RCC exhibited many

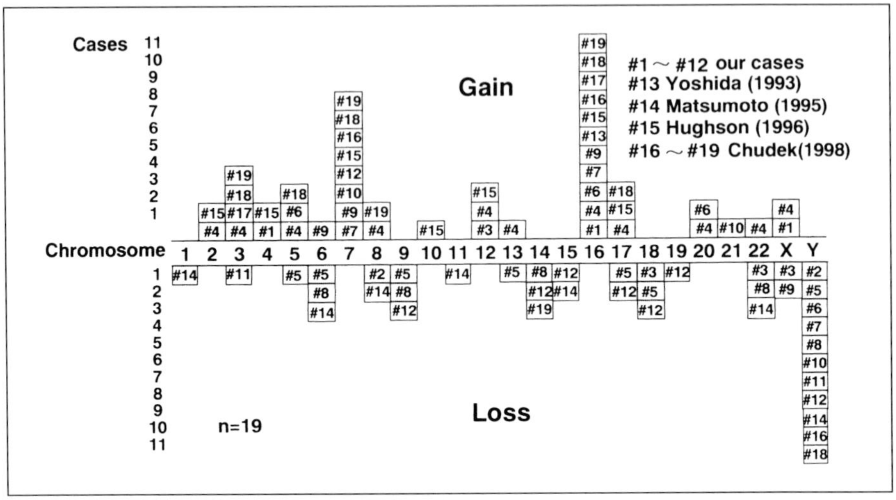

Fig. 5. Karyotypes of papillary renal cell carcinomas.

supernumerary chromosomes, mainly in chromosomes 12, 16 and X in 2 of 4 patients. Karyotypes of 7 additional cases of papillary RCC encountered in our institution were added to figure 5 including later studies [45–48]. The combined results revealed a relatively high incidence of trisomy 7 and 16 and loss of the Y chromosome (fig. 5). Three of four patients with nonpapillary RCCs revealed LOH at loci on 3p14 and 3p21 [44]. Hughson et al. [49] found a mutation of the von Hippel-Lindau (VHL) gene in 1 of 3 nonpapillary cancers. These karyotypic changes in papillary RCC and LOH on 3p in non-papillary RCC suggest that cytogenetic changes in RCC patients undergoing chronic hemodialysis are similar to those in nondialysis patients, although this conclusion is preliminary because the number of patients studied was small.

Pathogenesis of RCC in Dialysis Patients

The mechanism of RCC development in the atrophic kidneys with acquired cysts is very interesting both for clinicians and researchers; however, the etiology remains unclear [18]. One hypothesis is as follows, nephron loss causes hypertrophic changes and an unknown uremia-related growth factor develops. This causes tubular undifferentiated growth, genetic noise and an increased risk of mutation. Moreover, maturity-arrest immature tubular cells and a gene expression defect of the normal tubular structure exist and finally acquired cysts develop. Furthermore, the long-term effect of the uremia-related growth factor causes highly proliferative tubules finally resulting in an abnormality of separation of chromosomes or numerical change, as well as structural changes in chromosomes, followed by papillary or nonpapillary RCC. As double cancers were sometimes detected with RCC in dialysis patients, a common oncogene or impaired immune surveillance was also suggested as the cause of RCC development in dialysis patients.

No effective uremic animal model for RCC accompanied by acquired renal cystic disease has been developed. Some animal models have been reported, using N-ethyl-N-hydroxyethylnitrosamine with adenine [50], ferric agents nitriloacetate [51] and diphenylthiazole with N-nitrosomorpholine [52].

Diagnosis of RCC in Dialysis Patients

More than 90% of RCCs in dialysis patients do not show any symptoms. Symptoms include gross hematuria which is the most profound symptom, then followed by abdominal pain, fever, erythrocytosis, anemia, hypercalcemia or symptoms of metastasis. About 90% of RCC cases were found by imaging studies, either sonographic or computed tomographic (CT) examinations [9]. Protrusion of the solid mass from the contour of the kidney is a diagnostic aid for relatively short-term hemodialysis; however, RCC in long-term dialysis develops within the contour of the native kidney and is surrounded by multiple acquired cysts. If sonographic analysis reveals an echogenic mass, helical CT with bolus injection of contrast media is the next diagnostic procedure for RCC. Vascularity should be verified with this procedure, e.g. whether it is a hyper- or hypovascular tumor [6]. A mass without enhancement indicates hemorrhagic cysts. Dynamic CT or magnetic resonance (MR) is useful to make a final preoperative diagnosis [6, 53]. MR imaging can detect smaller tumors than sonography [54]. The differential diagnosis of hemorrhagic cysts is necessary when MR imaging is used [55]. Diagnoses of RCCs are clear after renal transplantation due to the regression of acquired renal cysts [43].

No tumor marker [56] is useful for the diagnosis of RCC in dialysis patients. In rare cases, the erythropoietin concentration may be a tumor maker. In very few patients is dialysis associated with pheochromocytoma [57]. This condition should be differentiated from RCC.

Screening for RCC in Dialysis Patients

Controversy remains regarding the need to screen for RCC in all dialysis patients. Ishikawa et al. [3, 6] recommended yearly screening because the frequency of RCC in Japan is high, many young long-term dialysis patients exist although few renal transplantations are performed, RCC is usually asymptomatic and some dialysis patients with RCC have metastases. Many studies have shown the value of screening patients on dialysis for more than 3 years [58, 59]. The screening rate for RCC is high in dialysis centers in Japan. However, Chandhoke et al. [60] reported that screening, using decision analysis, was unnecessary because the incidence of RCC was not high based on autopsy results and because they supported the theory that RCC is not related to acquired renal cystic disease. Death from renal malignancies does not appear to be greater for dialysis patients than for the nondialysis population. Sarasin et al. [61] compared 2 screening methods by decision analysis. With screening, the life span of a 20-year-old dialysis patient whose residual life span is 25 years may be prolonged by only 1.6 years. For a 58-year-old patient, beginning dialysis with a life expectancy of 5 years, screening may prolong the life expectancy by only 4 or 5 days. Therefore, they concluded that routine screening for all dialysis patients was not justified in terms of cost effectiveness. However, they supported screening patients with a high risk for RCC. At present, young male patients on long-term dialysis with enlarged kidneys due to acquired renal cystic disease should be screened yearly either by sonography or CT. Furthermore, all dialysis patients should be examined before renal transplantation.

Treatment of RCC in Dialysis Patients

The treatment of choice for RCC in dialysis patients is nephrectomy [6]. Nephrectomy is indicated for all tumors diagnosed by imaging. If a tumor reveals vascularity either by enhanced CT or MR and a hemorrhagic cyst is ruled out, all tumors should be removed by nephrectomy regardless of the tumor size. A tumor larger than 1 cm in diameter should be nephrectomized if it is diagnosed, because tumors sometimes show rapid growth although large numbers of tumors reveal slow growth.

Unfortunately no method to differentiate between slowly and rapidly growing tumors has been established. Nephrectomy is performed only on the side of the tumor. Uninephrectomy is performed by lumbar oblique incision and simple or radical nephrectomy is carried out depending on the stage of RCC. Recently, nephrectomy using endoscopic manipulations [62] has been performed. Interferon is rarely used without confirmation of the effectiveness [63].

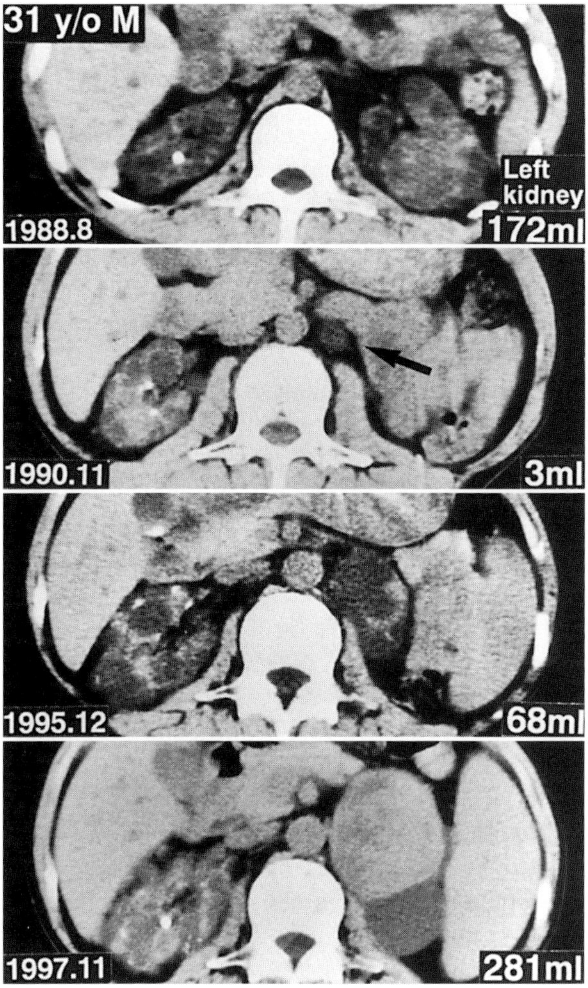

Fig. 6. CT findings 3, 7 and 9 years after left nephrectomy for renal cell carcinoma. Local recurrence of acquired cysts and renal cell carcinoma is observed. From Ishikawa et al. [72].

Prognosis of RCC in Dialysis Patients

Sixteen percent of the patients revealed metastasis [9]. Metastatic organs are the same as RCC in nondialysis patients. The 5-year survival rate is better in Japan compared to that in other countries. Recently, a number of metastatic RCC cases among dialysis and transplant patients have been reported [53, 64–72]. We encountered a unique case of local recurrence (fig. 6) [9]. The potentially invasive nature of such tumors is further illustrated by the observation of local recurrence of RCC which developed in a kidney with acquired renal cysts and was surgically removed by simple nephrectomy. Histological classification of the RCC was grade 2, granular cell subtype with tubulopapillary structure: pT2N0M0V0. Recurrence, 10 years after nephrectomy, was recognized by biannual CT. Figure 6a, which was presented previously, shows a 4.5-cm RCC in the left kidney in a 31-year-old male who received hemodialysis for 15 years due to chronic glomerulonephritis. Left nephrectomy was performed in 1988. Figure 6b reveals a 1-cm cyst in the left retroperitoneum 2 years later (in 1990) and a 1-cm solid mass in the cyst wall 7 years later (in 1995; fig. 6c). He refused operation at this time. Nine years later (in 1997; fig. 6d), the tumor and cyst had enlarged, and 10 years later (in 1998), surgery was performed. Pathology revealed acquired renal cystic disease; the mixed cell subtype and papillary pattern were the same as that 10 years before. Although no definitive evidence was found, dissemination (implantation) of tubular cells may have occurred from the original left kidney at the initial nephrectomy. It is not known whether tubular cells disseminating implanting from the original left kidney during surgery cause cystic change in vivo. Furthermore, whether simple nephrectomy is effective for low stages such as pT1 and pT2 is unclear.

In summary, the frequency of RCC in dialysis patients is high and the prevalence is 1.5%. This number increases by 4-fold in hemodialysis patients after more than 10 years. In Japan, questionnaire studies revealed a total of 1,451 RCCs in dialysis patients. The incidence or diagnostic rate of RCC depends on the rate of screening to detect RCC because almost all of these patients (91%) reveal no symptoms. Generalized metastasis is observed in 16% during mean follow-up of 1 year. Young male patients on long-term hemodialysis and enlarged kidneys due to acquired renal cysts are at risk of developing RCC. The high incidence of RCC in long-term dialysis patients results because the development of RCC is related to acquired cysts. The incidence and severity of acquired cysts increase in long-term dialysis patients. RCC in long-term hemodialysis patients is mainly RCC with acquired renal cystic disease in which the pathology is granular or the mixed cell subtype and tubular or the papillary structural type. These RCCs reveal numerous chromosomal changes. The development of RCC in long-term hemodialysis patients is related to cyst formation. Multistep progression from a renal cyst to atypical cyst, adenoma and finally RCC is presumed, although no direct evidence has been confirmed by molecular analysis.

References

1 Registry of Japanese Society for Dialysis Therapy: An overview of regular dialysis treatment in Japan (as of Dec. 31, 1997) (in Japanese). Jpn Soc Dial Ther, Nagoya, 1998.
2 Dunnill MS, Millard PR, Oliver D: Acquired cystic disease of the kidneys: A hazard of long-term intermittent maintenance haemodialysis. J Clin Pathol 1977;30:868–877.
3 Ishikawa I, Saito Y, Onouchi Z, Kitada H, Suzuki S, Kurihara S, Yuri T, Shinoda A: Development of acquired cystic disease and adenocarcinoma of the kidney in glomerulonephritic chronic hemodialysis patients. Clin Nephrol 1980;14:1–6.
4 Ishikawa I: Uremic acquired cystic disease of kidney. Urology 1985;26:101–108.
5 Grantham JJ, Levine E: Acquired cystic disease: Replacing one kidney disease with another. Kidney Int 1985;28:99–105.
6 Ishikawa I: Uremic acquired renal cystic disease: Natural history and complications. Nephron 1991;58:257–267.
7 Ishikawa I, Saito Y, Shikura N, Kitada H, Shinoda A, Suzuki S: Ten-year prospective study on the development of renal cell carcinoma in dialysis patients. Am J Kidney Dis 1990;16:452–458.
8 Ishikawa I: Re: Acquired cystic disease of the kidney: A management dilemma. J Urol 1993;149:1146–1148.
9 Ishikawa I: Renal cell carcinoma in chronic hemodialysis patients: A 1996 questionnaire study (in Japanese). Jpn J Dial Ther 1998;31:209–217.
10 Gardner KD Jr, Evan AP: Cystic kidneys: An enigma evolves. Am J Kidney Dis 1984;3:403–413.
11 MacDougall ML, Welling LW, Wiegmann TB: Renal adenocarcinoma and acquired cystic disease in chronic hemodialysis patients. Am J Kidney Dis 1987;9:166–171.
12 Levine E: Renal cell carcinoma in uremic acquired renal cystic disease: Incidence, detection, and management. Urol Radiol 1992;13:203–210.
13 Gentle DL, Mandell J, Jennings T: Renal cortical neoplasm in a child with dialysis-acquired cystic kidney disease. Urology 1996;47:254–255.
14 Mattoo TK, Greifer I, Geva P, Spitzer A: Acquired renal cystic disease in children and young adults on maintenance dialysis. Pediatr Nephrol 1997;11:447–450.
15 Ishikawa I, Onouchi Z, Saito Y, Tateishi K, Shinoda A, Suzuki S, Kitada H, Sugishita N, Fukuda Y: Sex differences in acquired cystic disease of the kidney on long-term dialysis. Nephron 1985;39:336–340.
16 Ishikawa I, Moncrief JW, Aguirre F, Brindley BW, Mott CL: Acquired cystic kidney disease in continuous ambulatory peritoneal dialysis patients; in Maekawa M, Nolph KD, Kishimoto T, Moncrief JW (eds): Machine Free Dialysis for Patient Convenience. 4th ISAO Official Satellite Symposium on CAPD, Osaka, ISAO Press, 1984, pp 131–133.
17 Ishikawa I, Yuri T, Kitada H, Shinoda A: Regression of acquired cystic disease of the kidney after successful renal transplantation. Am J Nephrol 1983;3:310–314.
18 Ishikawa I: Acquired cystic disease: Mechanisms and manifestations. Semin Nephrol 1991;11:671–684.
19 MacDougall ML, Welling LW, Wiegmann TB: Prediction of carcinoma in acquired cystic disease as a function of kidney weight. J Am Soc Nephrol 1990;1:828–831.
20 Ishikawa I: Acquired renal cystic disease and its complications in continuous ambulatory peritoneal dialysis patients. Perit Dial Int 1992;12:292–297.
21 Nishida Y, Yorioka N, Arita M, Harada S, Yano A, Hiromoto N, Yamakido M: Case report of a patient with bilateral renal cell carcinoma successfully maintained on continuous ambulatory peritoneal dialysis after bilateral nephrectomy. Int J Artif Organs 1997;20:213–216.
22 Ishikawa I, Ishii H, Shinoda A, Tateishi K, Ben A, Suzuki K, Tsugawa R: Renal cell carcinoma of the native kidney after renal transplantation: A case report and review of the literature. Nephron 1991;58:354–358.
23 Ishikawa I: Acquired cysts and neoplasms of the kidneys in renal allograft recipients; in Berlyne GM (ed): The Kidney Today. Contrib Nephrol. Basel, Karger, 1992, vol 100, pp 254–268.
24 Doublet JD, Peraldi MN, Gattegno B, Thibault P, Sraer JD: Renal cell carcinoma of native kidneys: Prospective study of 129 renal transplant patients. J Urol 1997;158:42–44.

25 Kliem V, Kolditz M, Behrend M, Ehlerding G, Pichlmayr R, Koch KM, Brunkhorst R: Risk of renal cell carcinoma after kidney transplantation. Clin Transplant 1997;11:255–258.
26 Sant GR, Ucci AA Jr: Acquired renal cystic disease and adenocarcinoma following renal transplantation: A current urologic perspective. Urol Int 1998;60:108–112.
27 Wiesel M, Carl S, Drehmer I, Hofmann WJ, Zeier M, Staehler G: Significance of RCC in hemodialyses patients compared to renal allograft recipients. Urologe A 1997;36:126–129.
28 Imanishi M, Kunikata S, Akiyama T, Kurita T: Study on the seven cases of malignant tumor after renal transplantation in our institution and statistic data of malignant tumor after renal transplantation in Japan (in Japanese). Ishoku 1996;31:100–107.
29 Riehl J, Schmitt H, Fritz A, Fuzesi L, Sieberth H-G: Renal oncocytoma of the native kidney after renal transplantation. Am J Nephrol 1998;18:160–163.
30 Horiguchi T, Ishikawa I: Immunohistochemical study in acquired cystic disease of the kidney – Expression of vimentin, epidermal growth factor, epidermal growth factor receptor and c-erb B2 gene product (in Japanese). Jpn J Nephrol 1993;35:797–807.
31 Khurana KK, Truong LD, Verani RR: Image analysis of proliferating cell nuclear antigen expression and immunohistochemical profiles in renal cell carcinoma associated with acquired cystic kidney disease: Comparison with classic renal cell carcinoma. Mod Pathol 1998;11:339–346.
32 Kovacs J, Zilahy M, Gomba S: Morphology of cystic renal lesions. Lectin and immuno-histochemical study. Acta Chir Hung 1997;36:176–178.
33 Sabo E, Misselevich I, Behar J, Nativ O, Boss JH: Cellular dysplasia in acquired cystic renal disease: Comparison of histomorphometrically gauged nuclear parameters in normal kidneys, renal cell carcinomas and acquired cystic kidneys. Neoplasma 1997;44:266–271.
34 Herrera GA: C-erb B-2 amplification in cystic renal disease. Kidney Int 1991;40:509–513.
35 Dinda AK, Mathur M, Guleria S, Saxena S, Tiwari SC, Dash SC: Heat shock protein (HSP) expression and proliferation of tubular cells in end stage renal disease with and without haemodialysis. Nephrol Dial Transplant 1998;13:99–105.
36 Ishikawa I: Renal cell carcinoma in chronic hemodialysis patients – A 1990 questionnaire study and review of past questionnaires (in Japanese). Jpn J Dial Ther 1991;24:493–497.
37 Ishikawa I, Kovacs G: High incidence of papillary renal cell tumours in patients on chronic haemodialysis. Histopathology 1993;22:135–139.
38 Ishikawa I, Shinoda A: Renal adenocarcinoma with or without acquired cysts in chronic hemodialysis patients. Clin Nephrol 1983;20:321–322.
39 Cofan F, Parra E, Sole M, Ricart MJ, Oppenheimer F, Campistol JM, Vilardell J, Carretero P: Renal oncocytoma in a long-term renal-transplant recipient. Nephrol Dial Transplant 1995;10: 560–562.
40 Suvarna SK, Ahuja M, Brown CB: Sarcomatoid renal cell carcinoma arising in hemodialysis-associated acquired cystic kidney disease presenting with disseminated bone marrow infiltration. Am J Kidney Dis 1994;24:581–585.
41 Ito F, Horita S, Yanagisawa H, Ryoji O, Onitsuka S, Okuda H, Nakazawa H, Toma H: Bellini's duct tumor associated with end stage renal disease: A case diagnosed by lectin immunohistochemistry. Acta Urol Jpn 1993;39:735–738.
42 Rahilly MA, Jenkins DAS, Carey FA: Urothelial neoplasia complicating acquired cystic kidney disease. Nephrol Dial Transpl 1992;7:1136–1138.
43 Ishikawa I, Shikura N, Ozaki M: Papillary renal cell carcinoma with numeric changes of chromosomes in a long-term hemodialysis patient: A karyotype analysis. Am J Kidney Dis 1993;21:553–556.
44 Ishikawa I, Ozaki M, Tominaga Y, Nakamura Y: Cytogenetic abnormalities in renal cell carcinomas associated with uremic acquired renal cystic disease. J Kanazawa Med Univ 1996;21:76–81.
45 Yoshida MA, Shishikura A, Ohshima H, Ikeuchi T: Cytogenetic analyses of renal cell carcinoma cells from a patient with chronic renal failure, acquired cystic disease of the kidney and a constitutional chromosome translocation (abstract). Prog 52nd Ann Meet Jpn Cancer Assoc, Sendai, 1993, p 208.
46 Matsumoto M, Sakamoto K, Kamura K, Hamano S, Hachisu T, Kenmochi T, Yamada H, Maeda H, Kashiwabara H, Hamaguchi K, Yamada K, Yokoyama T: A case of renal cell carcinoma of the left native kidney following renal transplantation (in Japanese). Isyoku 1995;30:605–610.

47 Hughson MD, Meloni AM, Silva FG, Sandberg AA: Renal cell carcinoma in an end-stage kidney of a patient with a functional transplant: Cytogenetic and molecular genetic findings. Cancer Genet Cytogenet 1996;89:65–68.
48 Chudek J, Herbers J, Wilhelm M, Kenck C, Bugert P, Ritz E, Waldman F, Kovacs G: The genetics of renal tumors in end-stage renal failure differs from those occurring in the general population. J Am Soc Nephrol 1998;9:1045–1051.
49 Hughson MD, Schmidt L, Zbar B, Daugherty S, Meloni AM, Silva FG, Sandberg AA: Renal cell carcinoma of end-stage renal disease: A histopathologic and molecular genetic study. J Am Soc Nephrol 1996;7:2461–2468.
50 Tsuda H, Matsumoto K, Iwase T, Nishida Y, Baba H: Enhanced neoplastic lesion development with adenine-induced experimental multicystic nephropathy by adenine – A model system for the analysis of renal tumor generation in long-term hemodialysis patients. Cancer Lett 1994;83:105–110.
51 Kondo A, Deguchi J, Okada S: Renal cysts and associated renal tumours in male ddY mice injected with ferric nitrilotriacetate. Virchows Arch 1995;427:91–99.
52 Ito F, Toma H, Yamaguchi Y, Nakazawa H, Onitsuka S, Hashimoto Y: A rat model of chemical-induced polycystic kidney disease with multistage tumors. Nephron 1998;79:73–79.
53 Levine E: Acquired cystic kidney disease. Radiol Clin North Am 1996;34:947–964.
54 Heinz-Peer G, Maier A, Eibenberger K, Grabenwoger F, Kreuzer S, Ba-Ssalamah A, Watschinger B, Lechner G: Role of magnetic resonance imaging in renal transplant recipients with acquired cystic kidney disease. Urology 1998;51:534–538.
55 John G, Semelka RC, Burdeny DA, Kelekis NL, Woosley JT, Kettritz U, Freeman JA: Renal cell cancer: Incidence of hemorrhage on MR images in patients with chronic renal insufficiency. J Magn Reson Imaging 1997;7:157–160.
56 Polenakovic M, Sikole A, Dzikova S, Polenakovic B, Gelev S: Acquired renal cystic disease and tumor markers in chronic hemodialysis patients. Int J Artif Organs 1997;20:96–100.
57 Asaka S, Takayama Y, Tagawa S, Ito Y, Yoshimura A, Masunaga T, Oiwake H, Shinozaki K, Takeda R: Pheochromocytoma in a long-term hemodialysis patient, discovered as an adrenal incidentaloma. Intern Med 1997;36:403–407.
58 Marple JT, MacDougall M, Chonko AM: Renal cancer complicating acquired cystic kidney disease. J Am Soc Nephrol 1994;4:1951–1956.
59 Shingleton WB, Blalock J, Clark J, Bigler SA: Renal cell carcinoma in native kidneys of patients with end stage renal disease. J Miss State Med Assoc 1998;39:86–89.
60 Chandhoke PS, Torrence RJ, Clayman RV, Rothstein M: Acquired cystic disease of the kidney: A management dilemma. J Urol 1992;147:969–974.
61 Sarasin FP, Wong JB, Levey AS, Meyer KB: Screening for acquired cystic kidney disease: A decision analytic perspective. Kidney Int 1995;48:207–219.
62 Takahashi S, Nozuki M, Usui K, Murayama T, Yumita S, Kurokawa Y, Sekino H: Laparoscopic nephrectomy in two hemodialysis patients with renal cancer (in Japanese). Jin to Touseki 1997;42: 259–262.
63 Soramoto S, Fujita K, Takenaka I: Renal cell carcinoma following long-term hemodialysis: A case report (in Japanese). Nishinihon J Urol 1992;54:1360–1362.
64 Griffin SC, Williams G: Metastatic hypernephroma from a native kidney after cadaver renal transplantation. Postgrad Med J 1985;61:471–472.
65 Thomson BJ, Allan PL, Winney RJ: Acquired cystic disease of kidney: Metastatic renal adenocarcinoma and hypercalcaemia. Lancet 1985;ii:502–503.
66 O'Donnell C, Cutner A, Williams G: Metastatic native renal carcinoma in renal transplant recipients. Nephrol Dial Transplant 1988;3:690–693.
67 Almirall J, Mallofre C, Campistol JM, Montoliu J, Ribalta T, Revert L: Metastatic renal cell carcinoma in a hemodialysis patient with acquired renal cystic disease. Nephron 1989;52:96–97.
68 Oliva TG, Molina MG: Metastatic malignant tumor in native kidney with acquired cystic disease after renal transplantation. Eur J Radiol 1990;11:154–155.
69 Lien Y-HH, Kam I, Shanley PF, Schroter GPJ: Metastatic renal cell carcinoma associated with acquired cystic kidney disease 15 years after successful renal transplantation. Am J Kidney Dis 1991;18:711–715.

70 Nakamoto T, Igawa M, Mitani S, Ueda M, Usui A, Usui T: Metastatic renal cell carcinoma arising in a native kidney of a renal transplant recipient. J Urol 1994;152:943–945.
71 Beckingham IJ, O'Rourke JS, Bishop MC, Ansell ID, Morgan AG, Blamey RW: The use of DNA typing to clarify the origin of metastatic carcinoma after renal transplantation. Transplant Int 1994; 7:379–381.
72 Ishikawa I, Saito Y, Nakazawa T, Shiroma K, Suzuki K: Local recurrence of renal cell carcinoma and acquired cysts 10 years after tumour nephrectomy. Nephrol Dial Transplant 1998;13:3236–3239.

Isao Ishikawa, MD, Division of Nephrology, Department of Internal Medicine,
Kanazawa Medical University, Uchinada, Kahoku, Ishikawa 920-0293 (Japan)
Tel. +81 76 286 2211, Fax +81 76 286 2786, E-Mail isikawai@kanazawa-med.ac.jp

Hino O (ed): Kidney Cancer. Recent Results of Basic and Clinical Research.
Contrib Nephrol. Basel, Karger, 1999, vol 128, pp 45–50

TSC1 and *TSC2* Gene Mutations in Human Kidney Tumors

Kazunori Kajino, Okio Hino

Department of Experimental Pathology, Cancer Insititute, Tokyo, Japan

TSC1 and *TSC2* Genes as Tumor Suppressors

Tuberous sclerosis (TSC) is one of the autosomal dominant systemic disorders associated with renal cell carcinoma (RCC). Cook et al. [1] reported that RCC was detected in 2.2% of TSC patients. TSC patients also develop seizures, mental retardation, and benign hamartomas such as renal angiomyolipoma (AML). As for the causative abnormality for TSC, the germline mutations of the *TSC1* or *TSC2* genes have been identified by positional cloning [2, 3]. Mutations of the *TSC1* or *TSC2* genes contribute to each half of familial TSC cases. Loss of heterozygosity (LOH) at the *TSC1* or *TSC2* loci is detected in the TSC-associated RCC and hamartomas [4–7], suggesting the role of these genes as tumor suppressors. In rats, mutations of the *Tsc2* gene, a rat homologue of human *TSC2*, play a causative role in RCC. Biallelic mutations of the *Tsc2* gene are found both in chemically induced RCC of the rat [8] and spontaneous RCC of the Eker rat which has a germline mutation of the *Tsc2* gene [9]. Overexpression of the exogenous *Tsc2* gene suppressed the neoplastic phenotype of rat RCC cells in vitro [10] and tumorigenicity in vivo [11]. Furthermore the transgene of the *Tsc2* suppressed RCC of the Eker rat [12] and this finding presented solid evidence to prove that the *Tsc2* functions as a tumor suppressor. As for the *TSC1* gene, a role as a tumor suppressor is also strongly suggested by the results of LOH analysis, but there is no molecular evidence to prove it at present.

Structure and Expression of the *TSC1* and *TSC2* Genes

The *TSC1* and *TSC2* genes are located in chromosomes 9q34 and 16p13.3, respectively. The 8.6-kb *TSC1* transcript is widely expressed and is particularly abundant in skeletal muscle [2]. The protein product, hamartin, consists of 1,164 amino acids with the calculated molecular mass being 130 kD. It has a single potential transmembrane domain near the N terminus and a coiled-coil region beginning at amino acid position 730 [2]. As for the *TSC2* gene, the transcript is 5.5 kb in size, and the 180-kD protein product, tuberin, consisting of 1,784 amino acids, is widely expressed. According to Wienecke et al. [13], tuberin is highly expressed in the brain, heart and kidney, all of which are commonly affected in TSC patients. There is a leucine zipper consensus near the N terminus and a region of homology to the GTPase-activating protein (GAP) for Rap1, which is a member of the superfamily of Ras-related proteins, near the C terminus [3]. The Drosophila homologs of *TSC1* and *TSC2* have recently been identified [14].

Proposed Functions of *TSC1* and *TSC2* Proteins

The molecular mechanism by which the *TSC2*/*Tsc2* gene functions as a tumor suppressor is not fully understood, but the relevant data have recently been accumulating. By using antisense oligonucleotides and Rat1 fibroblasts, Soucek et al. [15] clearly demonstrated that inhibition of *Tsc2* expression blocked the G0/G1 arrest caused by serum withdrawal and induced G1/S transition with the increase in cyclin D1 expression. Later, Soucek et al. [16], using the *Tsc2*-positive and -negative rat embryonic fibroblasts, reported that in *Tsc2*-negative cells the cyclin-dependent kinase (CDK) inhibitor p27 is mislocalized to the cytoplasm and degraded more rapidly than in *Tsc2*-positive cells. The molecular pathway leading to the abnormal processing of p27 in *Tsc2*-negative cells has not yet been determined, but their work provided strong evidence that the loss of *Tsc2* function disrupts p27 function, induces CDK2 activation, and accelerates the G1/S transition of the cells. Several other studies show that the *TSC2* product has Rap1 GAP activity, the dysfunction of which may lead to constitutive activation of Rap1 [17], or Rab5 GAP activity-modulating endocytosis [18], or the transactivating domain [19] or the activity of regulating AP-1 in Eker rat RCC [20] or the activity to modulate transcription mediated by steroid hormone receptor family members [21]. The *TSC1* gene was identified just one and a half years ago, and at present there is no report on the molecular function of the gene. Recently, van Slegtenhorst et al. [22] showed that the *TSC1* product and *TSC2* product associate physically in vivo and suggested that they function in the same complex rather than in separate pathways. Because TSC caused by a *TSC1* mutation and that caused by a *TSC2* mutation present similar phenotypes, it is likely that both genes are involved in an identical cellular pathway regulating the cell cycle.

TSC-Associated Renal Tumor

Stillwell et al. [23] reported that renal lesions in TSC patients occur with a frequency of 54% (51/95) when detected clinically, and up to 100% (15/15) following postmortem examination [23]. Most TSC-associated lesions are AML and/or cysts, but RCC, oncocytoma, or leiomyosarcoma also occur in TSC patients. The LOH of the *TSC1* or *TSC2* locus is confirmed in TSC-associated AML, and that of *TSC2* is more frequently seen than that of the *TSC1* [5–7]. RCC develops in 2.2% of TSC patients [1]. Bjornsson et al. [4] studied 6 TSC-associated RCC cases, and found LOH of the *TSC1* locus (9q34) in 2 cases and that of *TSC2* (16p13) in 1 case. Several differences between TSC-associated RCC and sporadic RCC are pointed out. Washecka and Hanna [24] reported that in 16 TSC-associated RCC cases, 7 (43%) were seen in bilateral kidneys, in contrast to the incidence of bilaterality of 1.8–3.8% in sporadic RCC. In the same study, the median age of the patients was 28 years, 30 years younger than that of sporadic RCC patients, and the male:female ratio was 3:16, with a reversal of that in sporadic RCC. Histologically, clear cell carcinoma was the most common cell type, but a tumor with high-grade sarcomatoid differentiation was also seen [4, 24]. Bjornsson et al. [4] showed that 4 of 6 TSC-associated RCC patients displayed strong immunoreactivity against HMB-45, a marker of melanocyte/neural crest derivation. HMB-45 is known to be expressed in AML [25], but is negative in sporadic RCC. The HMB-45 positivity of TSC-associated RCC suggested that they may be related to AML [4]. Recently Pea et al. [26] suggested that TSC-associated RCC may be less common than previously estimated because some malignant epithelioid AMLs have been interpreted as RCC, and that all reported RCC in TSC patients must be reevaluated (fig. 1).

Involvement of the *TSC1* and *TSC2* Genes in Sporadic Renal Tumor

The LOH of the *TSC2* locus is also detected in sporadic AML [6], but there is no report about abnormalities of the *TSC1* or *TSC2* genes in human sporadic RCC. Currently the functional loss of the *VHL* gene is thought to play a primary role in human RCC. However, for the establishment of cancer cells, multiple genetic or epigenetic abnormalities are required, and genes other than the *VHL* gene may be involved in the progression of RCC. Therefore we studied the LOH of the *TSC1* or *TSC2*, the rat homologue of which has been confirmed to function as the tumor suppressor for RCC, in sporadic human RCC cases. We obtained data showing that the LOH of the *TSC1* or *TSC2* genes was infrequent in sporadic RCC (mostly clear cell type), whereas 2 of 4 sporadic renal AML showed LOH of the *TSC2* gene (manuscript in preparation). The absence of LOH does not

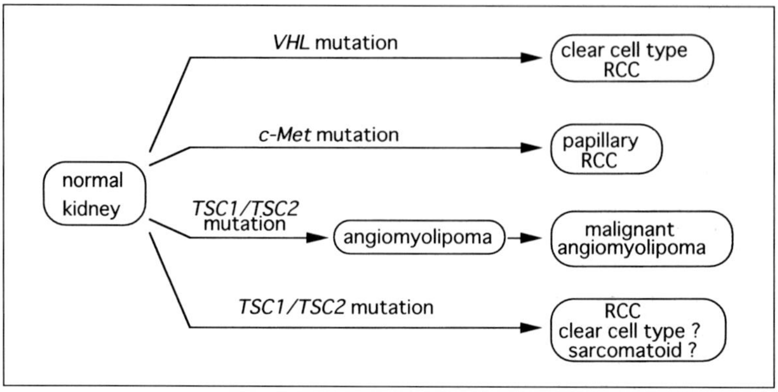

Fig. 1. Pathways of renal carcinogenesis.

completely deny the involvement of abnormal *TSC1*/*TSC2* in the process of human renal carcinogenesis, but it is less likely that they play a major role.

Cell Type-Specific, Species-Specific Tumorigenesis

Renal AML arises as the result of two hit mutations of the *TSC1*/*TSC2* genes, and most AMLs have a benign course [27]. The question is why the abnormality of rat *Tsc2* can cause RCC and that of human *TSC2* can cause benign AML in the same organ. There is no clear answer but several possibilities must be considered. First, it is known that human cells are generally more resistent to neoplastic transformation than rodent cells [28]. Second, p27 seems to play important roles in *Tsc2*-associated cell cycle regulation. The exact function or processing of p27 and related molecules may be different in human and rodent cells. Third, the species-specific modifier factors which epigenetically regulate tumor formation, such as the *Mom-1* [29, 30], may exist. Fourth, the cells in which the *TSC2*/*Tsc2* mutation occurs may be different in humans and rats. Or by unknown mechanisms, mutation of the gene more preferentially gives proliferating ability to the renal tubular cell in the rat, and to component cells of AML (vessels, muscle, or fat cells) in the human. Fifth, despite the histological difference, both rat RCC and human AML behave very similarly from the biological point of view. They do not metastasize or invade the adjacent organs, and cannot kill the host unless massive hemorrhage due to rupture occurs. Therefore, both of them may have some common molecular features specific to *TSC2*/*Tsc2* abnormality, although their morphological appearance is quite different. Sixth, experimental rats, including the Eker rat, are in most cases inbred. It is possible that experimental rats may have an accelerating factor for cancerization as a result of the pairing of an unknown recessive gene, which occurs very rarely in human cases. It should be interesting to mate the Eker rat with a wild, non-inbred rat and see if RCC appears in these rats or not.

Actually, a difference in tumor development between the original Eker rats (LE/LE) and F1 hybrid rats (LE/BN) is observed [31; Kikuchi et al., manuscript in preparation]. The data indicates that there is a modifier gene(s) in the BN rat genome that suppress the growth of tumors. Identification of such a modifier gene(s) might help to understand the species specificity or tumorigenicity of not only the *TSC2/Tsc2* mutation but also those of other tumor-suppressor genes.

Acknowledgment

This work was supported by the Organization for Pharmaceutical Safety and Research (OPSR).

References

1 Cook JA, Oliver K, Mueller RF, Sampson J: A cross sectional study of renal involvement in tuberous sclerosis. J Med Genet 1996;33:480–484.

2 van Slegtenhorst M, de Hoogt R, Hermans C, Nellist M, Janssen B, Verhoef S, Lindhout D, van den Ouweland A, Halley D, Young J, Burley M, Jeremiah S, Woodward K, Nahmias J, Fox M, Ekong R, Osborne J, Wolfe J, Povey S, Snell RG, Cheadle JP, Jones AC, Tachataki M, Ravine D, Sampson JR, Reeve MP, Richardson P, Wilmer F, Munro C, Hawkins TL, Sepp T, Ali JBM, Ward S, Green AJ, Yates JRW, Kwiatkowska J, Henske EP, Short MP, Haines JH, Jozwiak S, Kwiatkowski DJ: Identification of the tuberous sclerosis gene *TSC1* on chromosome 9q34. Science 1997;277:805–808.

3 The European Chromosome 16 Tuberous Sclerosis Consortium: Identification and characterization of the tuberous sclerosis gene on chromosome 16. Cell 1993;75:1305–1315.

4 Bjornsson J, Short MP, Kwiatkowski DJ, Henske EP: Tuberous sclerosis-associated renal cell carcinoma. Am J Pathol 1996;149:1201–1208.

5 Green AJ, Johnson PH, Yates JRW: The tuberous sclerosis gene on chromosome 9q34 acts as a growth suppressor. Hum Mol Genet 1994;3:1833–1834.

6 Henske EP, Neumann HPH, Scheithauer BW, Herbst EW, Short MP, Kwiatkowski DJ: Loss of heterozygosity in the tuberous sclerosis *(TSC2)* region of chromosome band 16p13 occurs in sporadic as well as TSC-associated renal angiomyolipomas. Genes Chromosomes Cancer 1995;13:295–298.

7 Carbonara C, Longa L, Grosso E, Mazzucco G, Borrone C, Garre ML, Brisigotti M, Filippi G, Scabar A, Giannotti A, Falzoni P, Monga G, Garini G, Gabrielli M, Riegler P, Danesino C, Ruggieri M, Magro G, Migone N: Apparant preferential loss of heterozygosity at *TSC2* over *TSC1* chromosomal region in tuberous sclerosis hamartomas. Genes Chromosomes Cancer 1996;15:18–25.

8 Satake N, Urakami S, Hirayama Y, Izumi K, Hino O: Biallelic mutations of the Tsc2 gene in chemically induced rat renal carcinoma. Int J Cancer 1998;77:895–900.

9 Kobayashi T, Urakami S, Hirayama Y, Yamamoto T, Nishizawa M, Takahara T, Kubo Y, Hino O: Intragenic *Tsc2* somatic mutations as Knudson's second hit in spontaneous and chemically induced renal carcinomas in the Eker rat model. Jpn J Cancer Res 1997;88:254–261.

10 Orimoto K, Tsuchiya H, Kobayashi T, Matsuda T, Hino O: Suppression of the neoplastic phenotype by replacement of the *Tsc2* gene in Eker rat renal carcinoma cells. Biochem Biophys Res Commun 1996;219:70–75.

11 Jin F, Wienecke R, Xiao GH, Maize JC Jr, DeClue JE, Yeung RS: Suppression of tumorigenicity by the wild-type tuberous sclerosis 2 *(Tsc2)* gene and its C-terminal region. Proc Natl Acad Sci USA 1996;93:9154–9159.

12 Kobayashi T, Mitani H, Takahashi R, Hirabayashi M, Ueda M, Tamura H, Hino O: Transgenic rescue from embryonic lethalty and renal carcinogenesis in the Eker rat model by introduction of a wild-type *Tsc2* gene. Proc Natl Acad Sci USA 1997;94:3990–3993.
13 Wienecke R, Maize JC Jr, Reed JA, de Gunzburg J, Yeung RS, DeClue JE: Expression of the *TSC2* product tuberin and its target Rap1 in normal human tissues. Am J Pathol 1997;150:43–50.
14 Ito N, Rubin GM: Gigas, a Drosophila homolog of tuberous sclerosis gene product-2, regulates the cell cycle. Cell 1999;96:529–539.
15 Soucek T, Pusch O, Wienecke, DeClue JE, Hengstschlager M: Role of the tuberous sclerosis gene-2 product in cell cycle control. J Biol Chem 1997;272:29301–29308.
16 Soucek T, Yeung RS, Hengstschlager M: Inactivation of the cyclin-dependent kinase inhibitor p27 upon loss of the tuberous sclerosis complex gene-2. Proc Natl Acad Sci USA 1998;95:15653–15658.
17 Wienecke R, Konig A, DeClue JE: Identification of tuberin, the tuberous sclerosis-2 product. J Biol Chem 1995;270:16409–16414.
18 Xiao G-H, Shoarinejad F, Jin F, Golemis EA, Yeung R: The tuberous sclerosis 2 gene product, tuberin, functions as a Rab5 GTPase activating proten (GAP) in modulating endocytosis. J Biol Chem 1997;272:6097–6100.
19 Tsuchiya H, Orimoto K, Kobayashi T, Hino O: Presence of potent transcriptional activation domains in the predisposing tuberous sclerosis (*Tsc2*) gene product of the Eker rat model. Cancer Res 1996;56:429–433.
20 Urakami S, Tsuchiya H, Orimoto K, Kobayashi T, Igawa M, Hino O: Overexpression of members of the AP-1 transcriptional factor family from an early stage of renal carcinogenesis and inhibition of cell growth by AP-1 gene antisense oligonucleotides in the *Tsc2* gene mutant (Eker) rat model. Biochem Biophys Res Commun 1996;241:24–30.
21 Henry KW, Yuan X, Koszewski NJ, Onda H, Kwiatkowski DJ, Noonan DJ: Tuberous sclerosis gene 2 product modulated transcription mediated by steroid hormone receptor family members. J Biol Chem 1998;273:20535–20539.
22 van Slegtenhorst, Nellist M, Nagelkerken B, Cheadle J, Snell R, van den Ouweland A, Reuser A, Sampson J, Halley D, van der Sluijs P: Interaction between hamartin and tuberin, the TSC1 and TSC2 gene products. Hum Mol Genet 1998;7:1053–1057.
23 Stillwell TJ, Gomez MR, Kelalis PP: Renal lesions in tuberous sclerosis. J Urol 1987;138:477–481.
24 Washecka R, Hanna M: Malignant renal tumors in tuberous sclerosis. Urology 1991;37:340–343.
25 Pea M, Bonetti F, Zamboni G, Martignoni G, Riva M, Colombari R, Mombello A, Bonzanini M, Scarpa A, Ghimenton C, Donati LF: Melanocyte-marker-HMB-45 is regularly expressed in angiomyolipoma of the kidney. Pathology 1991;23:185–188.
26 Pea M, Bonetti F, Martignoni G, Henske EP, Manfrin E, Colato C, Bernstein J: Apparant renal cell carcinoma in tuberous sclerosis are heterogeneous: The indication of malignant epithelioid angiomyolipoma. Am J Surg Pathol 1998;22:180–187.
27 Zimmerhackl LB, Rehm M, Kaufmehl K, Kurlemann G, Brandis M: Renal involvement in tuberous sclerosis complex: A retrospective survey. Pediatr Nephrol 1994;8:451–457.
28 Holliday R: Neoplastic transformation: The contrasting stability of human and mouse cells; in Lindahl T (ed): Genetic Instability in Cancer. New York, Cold Spring Harbor Laboratory Press, 1996, pp 103–115.
29 Dietrucg WF, Lander ES, Smith JS, Moser AR, Gould KA, Luoungo C, Borenstein N, Dove W: Genetic dentification of *Mom-1*, a major modifier locus affecting *Min*-induced intestinal neoplasia in the mouse. Cell 1993;75:631–639.
30 MacPhee M, Chepenik KP, Liddell RA, Nelson KK, Siracusa LD, Buchberg AM: The secretory phospholipase A2 gene is a candidate for the *Mom1* locus, a major modifier of Apc^{Min}-induced intestinal neoplasia. Cell 1995;81:957–966.
31 Hino O, Satake N, Kobayashi T, Kajino K: Carcinogenesis in tuberous sclerosis. Gann Monogr Cancer Res 1999;46:101–111.

Okio Hino, MD, PhD, Department of Experimental Pathology, Cancer Institute,
1-37-1, Kami-Ikebukuro, Toshima-ku, Tokyo 170-8455 (Japan)
Tel./Fax +81 3 5394 3815, E-Mail ohino@ims.u-tokyo.ac.jp

Hino O (ed): Kidney Cancer. Recent Results of Basic and Clinical Research.
Contrib Nephrol. Basel, Karger, 1999, vol 128, pp 51–61

Classification of Renal Cell Cancer Based on (Cyto)genetic Analysis

Eva van den Berg, Trijnie Dijkhuizen

Department of Medical Genetics, University of Groningen, The Netherlands

Introduction

Renal cell cancer (RCC) is a heterogeneous group of tumors and represents 85% of all primary renal neoplasms in adults, effecting males twice as often as females. The overall incidence increases with each decade of life, showing a peak in the sixth decade [1, 2]. In rare instances, RCC also affects children and young adults [3–5]. There is no clear geographical or ethnic preference, although there is a higher incidence in Scandinavia and the United States [3]. An increased incidence of RCC has been described in patients with end-stage renal disease or patients with acquired cystic kidney disease [6–8]. Also, environmental factors like smoking, obesity and occupational exposure increase the risk of RCC [9]. RCCs are often quite large at detection and already have metastasized. At present there is no effective therapy for metastatic RCC and patients with irresectable disease have a poor prognosis [2, 3].

Clinicopathologically, RCC consists of a number of histologically defined entities which may occur either nonhereditarily or hereditarily. This heterogeneity is a well-known complicating factor in the diagnosis. The histogenesis of RCC has been controversial for a long time, especially in terms of the thesis originally expressed by Virchow and advocated by Grawitz [10] that certain clear cell epithelial renal tumors are derived from ectopic adrenocortical elements. This has led to the term 'hypernephroma' or Grawitz tumor. Nowadays, there is evidence that the usual (nonembryonic) RCC in all its variants derives, in principle, from the mature uriniferous tubule. This is based also on animal experiments and observation of pre-stages and early stages of epithelial renal tumors in human kidneys [11, 12].

Morphologic Histologic Classification of Renal Cell

The aim of a histopathological classification to identify biologically distinct groups of RCC is, on the basis of morphological criteria, the recognition of which are of clinical value [13].

Currently several morphological classifications are used: one according to the WHO/AFIP [12] and one according to Störkel et al. [14] (modification of the Mainz classification [15, 16], as well as the Heidelberg classification by Kovacs et al. [17]). As stated in the latter two, eight different subtypes of RCC can be distinguished, related to the basic cell types of the nephron from which they are derived and in line with the genetic facts as presently understood: (1) metanephric adenoma and metanephric adenofibroma; (2) papillary adenoma, and (3) renal oncocytoma. All three are benign parenchymal neoplasms. Malignant parenchymal neoplasms are: (4) common or conventional (clear cell) renal carcinoma; (5) papillary (formerly chromophilic or tubulopapillary) renal carcinoma; (6) chromophobe renal carcinoma; (7) collecting duct carcinoma, and (8) renal cell carcinoma, unclassified. These types show phenotypical/histogenetical relations to different parts of cell types, respectively, of the nephron collecting duct system [14, 17].

(Molecular) Cytogenetic and Morphologic Correlations

Cytogenetics allow the classification of tumors with respect to their genotypic differences. Figure 1 summarizes and correlates both morphology and cytogenetic data with respect to histogenetic aspects of most of the basic tumor subtypes mentioned above.

Metanephric adenoma or adenofibroma are not included in figure 1 because of the limited data available: a study of 11 cases by fluorescent in situ hybridization identified gain of chromosomes 7 and 17 with Y chromosome loss suggesting a relationship with papillary renal cell adenomas and carcinomas [18]. The only cytogenetic study reported so far revealed a normal karyotype [19].

Most papillary renal adenomas and carcinomas are characterized by a unique combination of autosomal trisomies with trisomy 17 as the most frequent finding. Papillary adenomas specifically show a –Y, +7, +17 chromosomal pattern as well as trisomy 3 or gain of the long arm of chromosome 3 [20–26], although the latter finding probably reflects malignant transformation [21]. The high incidence of loss of the Y chromosome combined with the strong male preponderance suggests that loss of specific sequences harbored on the Y chromosome probably are important for developing this subtype.

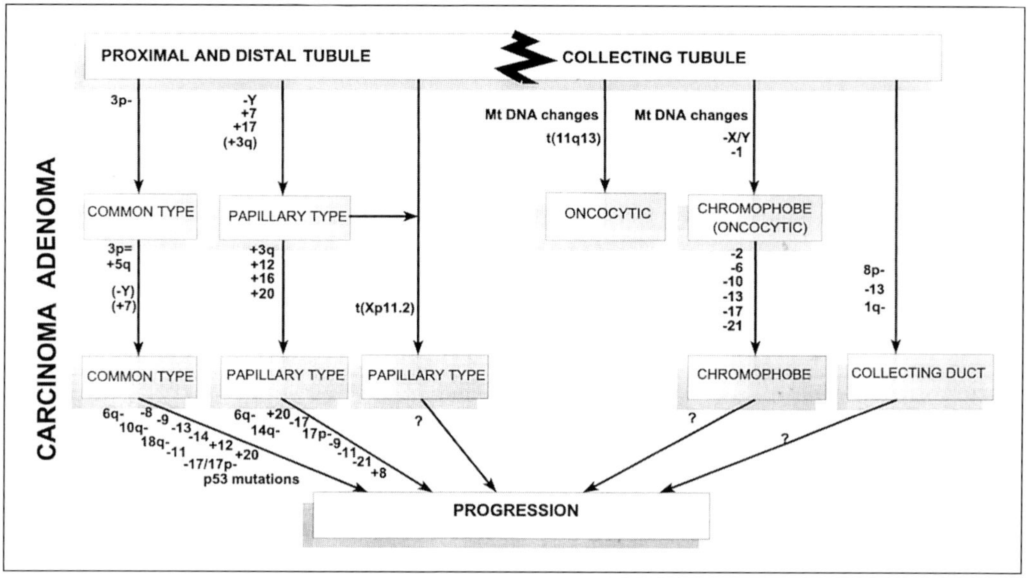

Fig. 1. Revised proposed oncogenetic model for renal cell cancer.

Also, the incidence of trisomy 7 is substantially higher than observed in apparently normal kidney tissue and therefore considered an essential step in the oncogenesis of papillary tumors [25, 26].

Trisomy of chromosomes 12, 16, 20 is associated with progression from the adenoma into the carcinoma stage, i.e. papillary renal cell carcinomas [25–29]. No mutations of p53 have been observed in this subtype, suggesting that the p53 gene most likely does not play an important role [26]. Palmedo et al. [25, 30] reported allelic duplications of 7q31–33, 17q12–22, 16q24–qter, 12q12–14, 8p21, 3q22–24, at 20q11.2 and 20q13.2 by microsatellite analysis. The latter finding probably marking new tumor genes in papillary renal carcinoma. The MET proto-oncogene, assigned to 7q31 and that encodes the receptor for hepatocyte growth factor/scatter factor implicated in the proliferation and invasiveness, is also involved in germline and somatic mutations in papillary renal tumors [31–33]. Cytogenetically, no differences are observed between hereditary tumors (usually presenting as multiple/bilateral tumors, and especially in familiar cases characterized by an early age of onset) and sporadic papillary tumors [3].

A small subset of papillary RCC is characterized by X; 1 autosome translocations [34]. The t(X; 1)(p11.2; q21) appears to be a specific primary anomaly, suggesting that tumors with this translocation form a distinct subgroup of papillary RCCs, showing clear cell cytoplasma. These tumors occur in young adults and children, preferentially in male patients although female cases have recently been described [4, 35–42]. The genes involved in the t(X; 1)(p11.2; q21) have been cloned [43, 44] and it has been shown that the translocation results in a fusion of the transcription factor TFE3 on the X chromosome, with a novel gene, designated PRCC, on chromosome 1 [45, 46].

The most frequent finding in common type renal carcinoma is loss of sequences of the short arm of chromosome 3 due to a deletion or unbalanced translocation [24, 29, 47–49]. In the dominantly inherited von Hippel-Lindau (VHL) cancer syndrome the VHL gene, assigned to 3p25, is mutated in the germ line and in renal cell tumors of affected family members [50]. This gene seems also to play a role in the development of the sporadic forms, probably in combintion with other gene(s) [51–54]. Other regions at 3p frequently found to be lost are 3p12–14 and 3p21. Moreover, van den Berg et al. [55, 56] showed that loss of at least two of the regions mentioned above are necessary for kidney cells to develop into common type renal cell carcinoma, and loss of 3p21 is obligatory (3p=; fig. 1). Tumors showing only one deletion at 3p (3p–; fig. 1), either 3p14 or 3p25, should be designated common type renal cell adenomas. The possible role of the fragile histidine trial (FHIT) gene, assigned to 3p14 is a matter of debate [56–59]. Also a candidate gene, nonpapillary renal cell carcinoma 1 (NRC-1) has been identified and mapped with 3p12 [60].

In familial cases with a constitutional balanced translocation involving 3p, the distal 3p segment is consistently lost in tumor tissue [3, 61]. Involvement of the long arm (3q) has also been described in sporadic and hereditary cases [23, 62, 63].

Also a (partial) trisomy of chromosome 5, especially the 5q22-qter segment [64], is frequently found in common RCC as well as trisomy 12 and 20, loss of chromosomes 8, 9, 13q, 14q, and structural abnormalities of the long arm of chromosomes 6 and 10 [29, 49, 53, 65–70].

Renal oncocytoma is characterized by mitochondrial DNA changes [71], a feature shared with the chromophobe renal cell carcinoma. Several subsets can be distinguished: one with mixed populations of normal and abnormal karyotypes without any cytogenetic similarity (yet); one specifically defined numerical anomalies, in particular loss of chromosomes 1 and Y/X [72–74], and a group defined by (variant) translocations involving 11q13 [75–77]. Recently Sinke et al. [78] mapped this oncocytoma specific 11q13 breakpoint between D11S433/D11S146 and the BCL 1 locus.

Loss of chromosomes 1 (in particular loss of 1p) and loss of Y/X probably results in loss of tumor suppressor gene(s) responsible for this subset of renal oncocytomas [74, 79, 80]. Also, loss of chromosome 14q has been described [74, 80].

Since loss of Y/X and 1 has also been observed in chromophobe renal cell carcinoma, oncocytomas showing –Y/–X,–1 might progress to chromophobe renal cell carcinomas through additional chromosome losses (fig. 1) [76], also explaining their occasionally malignant behavior.

Chromophobe renal carcinomas show multiple losses of entire chromosomes, i.e. loss of chromosomes 1, 2, 6, 10, 13, 17, 21, and the Y or X chromosome, leading to a low chromosome number. They also show quantitative as well as qualitative changes in mitochondrial DNA [73, 81–89].

Reported cytogenetic data from collecting duct carcinomas did not reveal consistent findings: monosomy 1, 6, 14, 15, and 22 in one case [90] and trisomies 7, 12, 16, 17, and 20 in the other [91]. Schönberg et al. [92] reported involvement of the short arm of chromosome 8 related to poor prognosis and loss of the long arm of chromosome 13, both in 3 of 6 cases. Loss of the long arm of chromosome 1, region 1q32.1–q32.2, appeared to be a consistent finding in collecting duct carcinoma [93].

(Molecular) Cytogenetics and Tumor Progression

Common and papillary RCCs (both derived from the proximal or distal tubule) share a number of secondary karyotypic changes: loss of 6q, 9, 11, 14q, 17p, and gain of chomosomes 12 and 20 associated with tumor progression [29, 49, 94]. This suggests that many of the tumor suppressor loci involved may be common to the etiology of both forms [95]. Sarcomatoid transformation in RCC represents the highest form of dedifferentiation [14, 17]. Sarcomatoid variants of RCC can in principle be derived from all the basic cell types. Cytogenetic data on sarcomatoid RCC are scarce. Grammatico et al. [96] reported a sole case of pleuric effusion of sarcomatoid RCC with structural abnormalities of chromosomes 1, 5, 16, and 19, and we [97] found losses of 3p, 4(q), 6q, 8p, 9, 13, 14, 17p, and gain of 5, 12, and 20. Jiang et al. [98] reported gains of chromosomes 17 and 8q as well as losses of 13q, and 4q. We and others have found a relation between p53 mutations and sarcomatoid RCC [97, 99].

Cytogenetics Associated with Normal Kidney Tissue

Increasing evidence exists on the presence of clonal, mostly numerical, chromosomal changes in apparently normal kidney tissue from patients with a normal constitutional karyotype [100–104] like trisomy 5, 7, 8, 10, 18, and loss of the Y chromosome.

These changes are not an in vitro artefact and are independent of the length of cell culture [100]. Trisomy 7 and 10 and loss of the Y chromosome are also observed in renal cell tumors, raising the question whether these cells in the kidney have some inherent propensity for neoplasic transformation. Trisomy 7 has been proposed to represent the first oncogenetic step in the development of renal cancer. However, several tumors genetically revealing 3p deletions, do not exhibit trisomy 7. It has been shown that approximately 10% of kidney cells have trisomy 7 and neoplastic transformation occurs at similar frequencies in cells with and without trisomy 7 [105]. The presence of clonal and nonclonal aberrations in apparently normal kidney tissue merely indicates a chromosome instability pattern or mosaicism, and this condition should not be considered as strictly neoplastic.

Conclusion

Renal cell cancers are epithelial neoplasms that demonstrate a diversity of morphologic characteristics and clinical manifestations. Different subtypes of renal cell carcinoma might originate from cells of the different parts of the renal tubule. Taken together, cytogenetic and molecular genetic studies of recent years have demonstrated that certain specific chromosomal abnormalities correlate with different histological subtypes of RCC and could have diagnostic and prognostic consequences [70, 106, 107]. At the (cyto)genetic level, a (revised) proposed oncogenetic model for RCC is depicted in figure 1.

Thus, (cyto)genetic studies of renal adenomas, various subtypes of carcinomas and oncocytomas, will contribute to a better understanding of the biology of these tumors, and reveal key information on the process of tumorigenesis and tumor behavior.

References

1 Weiss LM, Gelb AB, Medeiros LJ: Adult renal epithelial neoplasms. Am J Clin Pathol 1995;103: 624–635.
2 Motzer RJ, Bander NH, Nanus DM: Renal cell carcinoma. N Engl J Med 1996;335:865–875.
3 Sandberg AA, Meloni-Ehrig AM: Renal cancer: Genetic and cytogenetic aspects; in Bertino JR (ed): Encyclopedia of Cancer. San Diego, Academic Press, 1997, vol III, pp 1522–1540.
4 de Jong B, Molenaar IM, Leeuw JA, Idunberg VJ, Oosterhuis JW: Cytogenetics of a renal adenocarcinoma in a 2-year-old child. Cancer Genet Cytogenet 1986;21:165–169.
5 Pedersen RK, Faurskov B, Hejl M, Kerndrup GB: Chromosome alterations in renal cell carcinoma of childhood may correspond to aberrations in adults. Cancer Genet Cytogenet 1998;106:166–169.
6 Bjornsson J, Short MP, Kwiatkowski DJ, Henske EP: Tuberous sclerosis-associated renal cell carcinoma – Clinical, pathological, and genetic features. Am J Pathol 1996;149:1201–1208.

7 Hughson MD, Schmidt L, Zbar B, Daugherty S, Meloni AM, Silva FG, Sandberg AA: Renal cell carcinoma of end-stage renal disease: A histopathologic and molecular genetic study. J Am Soc Nephrol 1996;7:2461–2468.
8 Kovacs G: High frequency of papillary renal-cell tumours in end-stage kidneys: Is there a molecular genetic explanation? Nephrol Dial Transplant 1995;10:593–596.
9 Mandel JS, McLaughlin JK, Schlehofer B, Mellemgaard A, Helmert U, Lindblad P, McCredie M, Adami HO: International renal-cell cancer study. 4. Occupation. Int J Cancer 1995;61:601–605.
10 Grawitz P: Die sogenannten Lipome der Niere. Virchows Arch [A] 1883;93:39–45.
11 Bannasch P, Zerban H: Animal models and renal carcinogenesis; in Eble JN (ed): Tumors and Tumor-Like Conditions of the Kidneys and Ureters. New York, Churchill Livingstone, 1990, pp 1–34.
12 Murphy WM, Beckwith JB, Farrow GM: Tumors of the kidney, bladder, and related urinary structures. Washington, Armed Forces Institute of Pathology, 1994.
13 Fleming S: The impact of genetics on the classification of renal carcinoma. Histopathology 1993; 22:89–92.
14 Storkel S, Eble JN, Adlakha K, Amin M, Blute ML, Bostwick DG, Darson M, Delahunt B, Iczkowski K: Classification of renal cell carcinoma: Workgroup No 1. Union Internationale Contre Le Cancer (UICC) and the American Joint Committee on Cancer (AJCC). Cancer 1997;80:987–989.
15 Thoenes W, Storkel S, Rumpelt HJ: Histopathology and classification of renal cell tumors (adenomas, oncocytomas and carcinomas). The basic cytological and histopathological elements and their use for diagnostics. Pathol Res Pract 1986;181:125–143.
16 Storkel S, van den Berg E: Morphological classification of renal cancer. World J Urol 1995;13: 153–158.
17 Kovacs G, Akhtar M, Beckwith BJ, Bugert P, Cooper CS, Delahunt B, Eble JN, Fleming S, Ljungberg B, Medeiros LJ, Moch H, Reuter VE, Ritz E, Roos G, Schmidt D, Srigley JR, Storked S, van den Berg E, Zbar B: The Heidelberg classification of renal cell tumours. J Pathol 1997;183:131–133.
18 Brown JA, Anderl KL, Borell TJ, Qian J, Bostwick DG, Jenkins RB: Simultaneous chromosome 7 and 17 gain and sex chromosome loss provide evidence that renal metanephric adenoma is related to papillary renal cell carcinoma. J Urol 1997;158:370–374.
19 Jones EC, Pins M, Dickersin GR, Young RH: Metanephric adenoma of the kidney: A clinicopathological, immunohistochemical, flow cytometric, cytogenetic, and electron microscopic study of seven cases. Am J Surg Pathol 1995;19:615–626.
20 Lager DJ, Huston BJ, Timmerman TG, Bonsib SM: Papillary renal tumors: Morphologic, cytochemical and genotypic features. Cancer 1995;76:669–673.
21 Kovacs G: Molecular cytogenetics of renal cell tumors. Adv Cancer Res 1993;62:89–124.
22 Renshaw AA, Fletcher JA: Trisomy 3 in renal cell carcinoma. Mod Pathol 1997;10:481–484.
23 Balzarini P, Dal Cin P, Roskams T, Polito P, Van Poppel H, Van Damme B, Baert L, Van den Berghe H: Histology may depend on the presence of partial monosomy or partial trisomy 3 in renal cell carcinoma. Cancer Genet Cytogenet 1998;105:6–10.
24 Hughson MD, Dickman K, Bigler SA, Meloni AM, Sandberg AA: Clear-cell and papillary carcinoma of the kidney: An analysis of chromosome 3, 7, and 17 abnormalities by microsatellite amplification, cytogenetics, and fluorescence in situ hybridization. Cancer Genet Cytogenet 1998; 106:93–104.
25 Palmedo G, Fischer J, Kovacs G: Fluorescent microsatellite analysis reveals duplication of specific chromosomal regions in papillary renal cell tumors. Lab Invest 1997;77:633–638.
26 Dijkhuizen T, van den Berg A, van den Berg E, Storkkel S, de Jong B, Seitz G, Henn W: Chromosomal findings and p53 mutation analysis in chromophilic renal cell carcinomas. Int J Cancer 1996;68: 47–50.
27 Henn W, Zwergel T, Wullich B, Thonnes M, Zang KD, Seitz G: Bilateral multicentric papillary renal tumors with heteroclonal origin based on tissue-specific karyotype instability. Cancer 1993; 72:1315–1318.
28 Kovacs G, Fuzesi L, Emannuel A, Kung H-F: Cytogenetics of papillary renal cell tumors. Gene Chromosome Cancer 1991;3:249–255.
29 van den Berg E, Dijkhuizen T, Oosterhuis JW, Geurts van Kessel A, de Jong B, Storkel S: Cytogenetic classification of renal cell cancer. Cancer Genet Cytogenet 1997;95:103–107.

30 Palmedo G, Fischer J, Kovacs G: Duplications of DNA sequences between loci D20S478 and D20S206 at 20q11.1 and between loci D20S902 and D20S480 at 20q13.2 mark new tumor genes in papillary renal cell carcinoma. Lab Invest 1999;79:311–316.
31 Schmidt L, Duh FM, Chen F, Kishida T, Glenn G, Choyke P, Scherer SW, Zhuang Z, Lubensky I, Dean M, Allikmets R, Chidambaram A, Bergerheim UR, Feltis JT, Casadevall C, Zamarron A, Bernues M, Richard S, Lips CJ, Walther MM, Tsui LC, Geil L, Orcutt ML, Stackhouse T, Zbar B, et al: Germline and somatic mutations in the tyrosine kinase domain of the MET proto-oncogene in papillary renal carcinomas. Nat Genet 1997;16:68–73.
32 Schmidt L, Junker K, Nakaigawa N, Kinjerski T, Weirich G, Miller M, Lubensky I, Neumann HP, Brauch H, Decker J, Vocke C, Brown JA, Jenkins R, Richard S, Bergerheim U, Gerrard B, Dean M, Linehan WM, Zbar B: Novel mutations of the MET proto-oncogene in papillary renal carcinomas. Oncogene 1999;18:2343–2350.
33 Glukhova L, Goguel AF, Chudoba I, Angevin E, Pavon C, Terrier-Lacombe MJ, Meddeb M, Escudier B, Bernheim A: Overrepresentation of 7q31 and 17q in renal cell carcinomas. Gene Chromosome Cancer 1998;22:171–178.
34 Dijkhuizen T, van den Berg E, Wilbrink M, Weterman M, Geurts van Kessel A, Storkel S, Folkers RP, Braam A, de Jong B: Distinct Xp11.2 breakpoints in two renal cell carcinomas exhibiting X; autosome translocations. Gene Chromosome Cancer 1995;14:43–50.
35 Tomlinson GE, Nisen PD, Timmons CF, Schneider NR: Cytogenetics of a renal cell carcinoma in a 17-month-old child: Evidence for Xp11.2 as a recurring breakpoint. Cancer Genet Cytogenet 1991;57:11–17.
36 Meloni AM, Sandberg AA, Pontes JE, Dobbs RM: Translocation (X; 1)(p11.2; q21): A subtype of renal adenocarcinomas. Cancer Genet Cytogenet 1992;63:100–101.
37 Meloni AM, Dobbs RM, Pontes JE, Sandberg AA: Translocation (X-1) in papillary renal cell carcinoma: A new cytogenetic subtype. Cancer Genet Cytogenet 1993;65:1–6.
38 Shipley JM, Birdsall S, Clark J, Crew J, Gill S, Linehan M, Gnarra J, Fisher S, Craig IW, Cooper CS: Mapping the X chromosome breakpoint in two papillary renal cell carcinoma cell lines with a t(X; 1)(p11.2; q21.2) and the first report of a female case. Cytogenet Cell Genet 1995;71: 280–284.
39 Kardas I, Denis A, Babinska M, Gronwald J, Podolski J, Zajaczek S, Kram A, Lubinski J, Limon J: Translocation (X; 1)(p11.2; q21) in a papillary renal cell carcinoma in a 14-year-old girl. Cancer Genet Cytogenet 1998;101:159–161.
40 Dal Cin P, Stas M, Sciot R, De Wever I, Van Damme B, Van Den Berghe H: Translocation (X; 1) reveals metastasis 31 years after renal cell carcinoma. Cancer Genet Cytogenet 1998;101:58–61.
41 Yenamandra A, Zhou XT, Trinchitella L, Susin M, Sastry S, Mehta L: Renal cell carcinoma with X; 1 translocation in a child with Klinefelter syndrome. Am J Med Genet 1998;77:281–284.
42 Perot C, Bougaran J, Boccon Gibod L, Storkel S, Leverger G, van den Akker J, Taillemite JL, Couturier J: Two new cases of papillary renal cell carcinoma with t(X; 1)(p11; q21) in females. Cancer Genet Cytogenet 1999;59:2021–2050.
43 Weterman MAJ, Wilbrink M, Janssen I, Janssen HAP, van den Berg E, Fisher SE, Craig I, Geurts van Kessel A: Molecular cloning of the papillary renal cell carcinoma-associated translocation (X; 1)(p11; q21) breakpoint. Cytogenet Cell Genet 1996;75:2–6.
44 Weterman M, Wilbrink M, Dijkhuizen T, van den Berg E, Geurts van Kessel A: Fine mapping of the 1q21 breakpoint of the papillary renal cell carcinoma-associated (X; 1) translocation. Hum Genet 1996;98:16–21.
45 Weterman MAJ, Wilbrink M, Geurts van Kessel A: Fusion of the transcription factor TFE3 gene to a novel gene: PPCC, in the t(X; 1)(p11; q21)-positive papillary renal cell carcinomas. Proc Natl Acad Sci USA 1996;93:15294–15298.
46 Sidhar SK, Clark J, Gill S, Hamoudi R, Crew AJ, Gwilliam R, Ross M, Linehan WM, Birdsall S, Shipley J, Cooper CS: The t(X; 1)(p11.2; q21.2) translocation in papillary renal cell carcinoma fuses a novel gene PRCC to the TFE3 transcription factor gene. Hum Mol Genet 1996;5:1333–1338.
47 Kovacs G, Wilkens L, Papp T: Nondisjunction reduplication of chromosome 3 is not a common mechanism in the development of human renal cell tumors. Cytogenet Cell Genet 1988;48:242–243.

48 van der Hout AH, van den Berg E, Van der Vlies P, Dijkhuizen T, Storkel S, Oosterhuis JW, de Jong B, Buys CHCM: Loss of heterozygosity at the short arm of chromosome-3 in renal-cell cancer correlates with the cytological tumour type. Int J Cancer 1993;53:353–357.
49 van den Berg E, van der Hout AH, Oosterhuis JW, Storked S, Dijkhuizen T, Dam A, Zweers HMM, Mensink HJA, Buys CHCM, de Jong B: Cytogenetic analysis of epithelial renal-cell tumors: Relationship with a new histopathological classification. Int J Cancer 1993;55:223–227.
50 Gnarra JR, Duan DR, Weng YK, Humphrey JS, Chen DYT, Lee S, Pause A, Dudley CF, Latif F, Kuzmin I, Schmidt L, Duh FM, Stackhouse T, Chen F, Kishida T, Wei MH, Lerman MI, Zbar B, Klausner RD, Linehan WM: Molecular cloning of the von Hippel-Lindau tumor suppressor gene and its role in renal carcinoma. Biochim Biophys Acta 1996;1242:201–210.
51 Whaley JM, Naglich J, Gelbert L, Hsia YE, Lamiell JM, Green JS, Collins D, Neumann HPH, Laidlaw J, Li FP, Klein-Szanto AJP, Seizinger BR, Kley N: Germ-line mutations in the von Hippel-Lindau tumor-suppressor gene are similar to somatic von Hippel-Lindau aberrations in sporadic renal cell carcinoma. Am J Hum Genet 1994;55:1092–1102.
52 Gnarra JR, Lerman MI, Zbar N, Linehan WM: Genetics of renal-cell carcinoma and evidence for a critical role for von Hippel-Lindau in renal tumorigenesis. Semin Oncol 1995;22:3–8.
53 Moch H, Schraml P, Bubendorf L, Richter J, Gasser TC, Mihatsch MJ, Sauter G: Intratumoral heterogeneity of von Hippel-Lindau gene deletions in renal cell carcinoma detected by fluorescence in situ hybridization. Cancer Res 1998;58:2304–2309.
54 Clifford SC, Prowse AH, Affara NA, Buys CHCM, Maher ER: Inactivation of the von Hippel-Lindau (VHL) tumour suppressor gene and allelic losses at chromosome arm 3p in primary renal cell carcinoma: Evidence for a VHL-independent pathway in clear cell renal tumourigenesis. Gene Chromosome Cancer 1998;22:200–209.
55 van den Berg A, Dijkhuizen T, Draaijers TG, Hulsbeek MMF, Maher ER, van den Berg E, Storkel S, Buys CHCM: Analysis of multiple renal cell adenomas and carcinomas suggests allelic loss at 3p21 to be a prerequiste for malignant development. Gene Chromosome Cancer 1997;19:228–232.
56 van den Berg A, Buys CHCM: Involvement of multiple loci on chromosome 3 in renal cell cancer development. Gene Chromosome Cancer 1997;19:59–76.
57 Huebner K, Garrison PN, Barnes LD, Croce CM: The role of the FHIT/FRA3B locus in cancer. Annu Rev Genet 1998;32:7–31.
58 Bugert P, Wilhelm M, Kovacs G: FHIT gene and the FRA3B region are not involved in the genetics of renal cell carcinomas. Gene Chromosome Cancer 1997;20:9–15.
59 Luan XD, Shi GP, Zohouri M, Paradee W, Smith DI, Decker HJ, Cannizzaro LA: The FHIT gene is alternatively spliced in normal kidney and renal cell carcinoma. Oncogene 1997;15:79–86.
60 Lott ST, Lovell M, Naylor SL, Killary AM: Physical and functional mapping of a tumor suppressor locus for renal cell carcinoma within chromosome 3p12. Cancer Res 1998;58:3533–3537.
61 Zbar B, Lerman M: Inherited carcinomas of the kidney. Adv Cancer Res 1998;75:163–201.
62 Koolen MI, van der Meyden PM, Bodmer D, Eleveld M, van der Looij E, Brunner H, Smits A, van den Berg E, Smeets D, Geurts van Kessel A: A familial case of renal cell carcinoma and a t(2; 3) chromosome translocation. Kidney Int 1998;53:273–275.
63 Bodmer D, Eleveld MF, Ligtenberg MJL, Weterman MAJ, Janssen BAP, Smeets DFCM, de Wit PEJ, van den Berg A, van den Berg E, Koolen MI, Geurts van Kessel A: An alternative route for multistep tumorigenesis in a novel case of hereditary renal cell cancer and a t(2; 3)(q35; q21) chromosome translocation. Am J Hum Genet 1998;62:1475–1483.
64 Bugert P, Von Knobloch R, Kovacs G: Duplication of two distinct regions on chromosome 5q in non-papillary renal-cell carcinomas. Int J Cancer 1998;76:337–340.
65 de Jong B, Oosterhuis JW, Idenburg VJ, Castedo SM, Dam A, Mensink HJ: Cytogenetics of 12 cases of renal adenocarcinoma. Cancer Genet Cytogenet 1988;30:53–61.
66 Presti JC, Rao PH, Chen Q, Reuter VE, Li FP, Fair WR, Jhanwar SC: Histopathological, cytogenetic, and molecular characterization of renal cortical tumors. Cancer Res 1991;51:1544–1552.
67 Meloni AM, Bridge J, Sandberg AA: Reviews on chromosome studies in urological tumors. 1. Renal tumors. J Urol 1992;148:253–265.
68 Maloney KE, Norman RW, Lee CLY, Millard OH, Welch JP: Cytogenetic abnormalities associated with renal cell carcinoma. J Urol 1991;146:692–696.

69 Schullerus D, Herbers J, Chudek J, Kanamaru H, Kovacs G: Loss of heterozygosity at chromosomes 8p, 9p, and 14q is associated with stage and grade of non-papillary renal cell carcinomas. J Pathol 1997;183:151–155.
70 Herbers J, Schullerus D, Muller H, Kenck C, Chudek J, Weimer J, Bugert P, Kovacs G: Significance of chromosome arm 14q loss in nonpapillary renal cell carcinomas. Gene Chromosome Cancer 1997;19:29–35.
71 Horton TM, Petros JA, Heddi A, Shoffner J, Kaufman AE, Graham SD, Gramlich T, Wallace DC: Novel mitochondrial DNA deletion found in a renal cell carcinoma. Gene Chromosome Cancer 1996;15:95–101.
72 Meloni AM, Sandberg AA, White RD: –Y, –1 as recurrent anomaly in oncocytoma. Cancer Genet Cytogenet 1992;61:108–109.
73 Crotty TB, Lawrence KM, Moertel CA, Bartelt DH, Batts KP, Dewald GW, Farrow GM, Jenkins RB: Cytogenetic analysis of 6 renal oncocytomas and a chromophobe cell renal carcinoma: Evidence that –Y, –1 may be a characteristic anomaly in renal oncocytomas. Cancer Genet Cytogenet 1992; 61:61–66.
74 Presti JC, Moch H, Reuter VE, Huynh D, Waldman FM: Comparative genomic hybridization for genetic analysis of renal oncocytomas. Gene Chromosome Cancer 1996;17:199–204.
75 van den Berg E, Dijkhuizen T, Storkel S, Brutel de la Riviere G, Dam A, Mensink HJ, Oosterhuis JW, de Jong B: Chromosomal changes in renal oncocytomas. Evidence that t(5; 11)(q35; q13) may characterize a second subgroup of oncocytomas. Cancer Genet Cytogenet 1995;79:164–168.
76 Dijkhuizen T, van den Berg E, Storkel S, de Vries B, van der Veen AY, Wilbrink M, Geurtz van Kessel A, de Jong B: Renal oncocytoma with t(5; 12; 11), der(1)t(1; 8) and add(19): 'True' oncocytoma or chromophobe adenoma? Int J Cancer 1997;73:521–524.
77 Neuhaus C, Dijkhuizen T, van den Berg E, Storkel S, Stockle M, Mensch B, Huber C, Decker HJ: Involvement of the chromosomal region 11q13 in renal oncocytoma: Case report and literature review. Cancer Genet Cytogenet 1997;94:95–98.
78 Sinke RJ, Dijkhuizen T, Janssen B, Olde Weghuis D, Merkx G, van den Berg E, Schuuring E, Meloni AM, de Jong B, Geurts van Kessel A: Fine mapping of the human renal oncocytoma-associated translocation (5; 11)(q35; q13) breakpoint. Cancer Genet Cytogenet 1997;96:95–101.
79 Trash-Bingham CA, Salazar H, Greenberg RE, Tartof KD: Loss of heterozygosity studies indicate that chromosome arm lp harbors a tumor suppressor gene for renal oncocytomas. Gene Chromosome Cancer 1996;16:64–67.
80 Herbers J, Schullerus D, Chudek J, Bugert P, Kanamaru H, Zeisler J, Ljungberg B, Akhtar M, Kovacs G: Lack of genetic changes at specific genomic sites separates renal oncocytomas from renal cell carcinomas. J Pathol 1998;184:58–62.
81 Kovacs A, Kovacs G: Low chromosome number in chromophobe renal cell carcinomas. Gene Chromosome Cancer 1992;4:267–268.
82 Speicher MR, Schoell B, du Manoir S, Schrock E, Ried T, Cremer T, Storkel S, Kovacs A, Kovacs G: Specific loss of chromosomes 1, 2, 6. 10, 13, 17, and 21 in chromophobe renal cell carcinomas revealed by comparative genomic hybridization. Am J Pathol 1994;145:356–364.
83 Shuin T, Kondo K, Sakai N, Kaneko S, Yao M, Nagashima Y, Kitamura H, Yoshida MA: A case of chromophobe renal cell carcinoma associated with low chromosome number and microsatellite instability. Cancer Genet Cytogenet 1996;86:69–71.
84 Gerharz CD, Moll R, Storkel S, Ramp U, Hildebrandt B, Molsberger G, Koldovsky P, Gabbert HE: Establishment and characterization of two divergent cell lines derived from a human chomophobe renal cell carcinoma. Am J Pathol 1995;146:953–962.
85 Marras S, Faa G, Scarpa R, Valdes E, Vanni R: Diagnosis of chromophobe renal cell carcinoma by chromosomal analysis. Tumori 1997;83:753–755.
86 Bugert P, Gaul C, Weber K, Herbers J, Akhtar M, Ljungberg B, Kovacs G: Specific genetic changes of diagnostic importance in chromophobe renal cell carcinomas. Lab Invest 1997;76:203–208.
87 Gunawan B, Bergmann F, Braun S, Hemmerlein B, Ringert RH, Jakse G, Fuzesi L: Polyploidization and losses of chromosomes 1, 2,6, 19, 13, and 17 in three cases of chromophobe renal cell carcinomas. Cancer Genet Cytogenet 1999;110:57–61.

88 Balzarini P, Grigolato P, Tardanico R, Cadei M, Cunico SC, Cozzoli A, Zanotelli T, Van Den Berghe H, Dal Cin P: Multitechnical pathological diagnosis in chromophobe renal cell carcinoma. Oncol Rep 1999;6:295–299.

89 Dijkhuizen T, van den Berg , Storkel S, de Jong B: Chromosome changes in a metastasis of a chromophobe renal cell tumor. Cancer Genet Cytogenet 1998;105:86–89.

90 Fuzesi L, Cober M, Mittermayer C: Collecting duct carcinoma: Cytogenetic characterization. Histopathology 1992;21:155–160.

91 Gregori-Romero MA, Morell-Quadreny L, Llombart-Bosch A: Cytogenetic analysis of three primary Bellini duct carcinomas. Gene Chromosome Cancer 1996;15:170–172.

92 Schoenberg M, Cairns P, Brooks JD, Marshall FF, Epstein JI, Isaacs WB, Sidransky D: Frequent loss of chromosome arms 8p and 13q in collecting duct carcinoma (CDC) of the kidney. Gene Chromosome Cancer 1995;12:76–80.

93 Steiner G, Cairns P, Polascik TJ, Marshall FF, Epstein JI, Sidransky D, Schoenberg MK: High-density mapping of chromosomal arm 1q in renal collecting duct carcinoma: Region of minimal deletion at 1q32.1–32.2. Cancer Res 1996;56:5044–5046.

94 Kovacs G: The value of molecular genetic analysis in the diagnosis of renal cell tumours. World J Urol 1994;12:64–68.

95 Thrash-Bingham CA, Greenberg RE, Howard S, Bruzel A, Bremer M, Goll A, Salazar H, Freed JJ, Tartof KD: Comprehensive allelotyping of human renal cell carcinomas using microsatellite DNA probes. Proc Natl Acad Sci USA 1995;92:2854–2858.

96 Grammatico P, Cianciulli AM, Grammatico B, Di Rosa C, Del Porto G: The first cytogenetic study of a sarcomatoid renal cell carcinoma. J Exp Clin Cancer Res 1993;12:19–21.

97 Dijkhuizen T, van den Berg E, van den Berg A, van de Veen A, Dam A, Faber H, Buys CHCM, Storkel S, de Jong B: Genetics as a diagnostic tool in sarcomatoid renal-cell cancer. Int J Cancer 1997;72:265–269.

98 Jiang F, Moch H, Riichter J, Egenter C, Gasser T, Bubendorf L, Gschwind R, Sauter G, Mihatsch MJ: Comparative genomic hybridization reveals frequent chromosome 13q and 4q losses in renal carcinomas with sarcomatoid transformation. J Pathol 1998;185:382–388.

99 Oda H, Nakatsuru Y, Ishikawa T: Mutations of the p53 gene and p53 protein overexpression are associated with sarcomatoid transformation in renal cell carcinomas. Cancer Res 1995;55:658–662.

100 Emanuel A, Szucs S, Weier HUG, Kovacs G: Clonal aberrations of chromosomes-X, Y, 7 and 10 in normal kidney tissue of patients with renal cell tumors. Gene Chromosome Cancer 1992;4:75–77.

101 Casalone R, Casalone PG, Minelli E, Portentoso P, Righi R, Meroni E, Giudici A, Donati D, Riva C, Salvatore S, Bono AV: Significance of the clonal and sporadic chromosome abnormalities in non-neoplastic renal tissue. Hum Genet 1992;90:71–78.

102 van den Berg E, Dijkhuizen T, Storkel S, Molenaar WM, de Jong B: Chromosomal abnormalities in non-neoplastic renal tissue. Cancer Genet Cytogenet 1995;85:152–154.

103 Knuutila S, Larramendy ML, Elfving P, El-Rifai W, Miettinen A, Mitelman F: Trisomy 7 in non-neoplastic tubular epithelial cells of the kidney. Hum Genet 1995;95:149–156.

104 Elfving P, Cigudosa JC, Lundgren R, Limon J, Mandahl N, Kristoffersson U, Heim S, Mitelman F: Trisomy 7, trisomy 10, and loss of the Y chromosome in short-term cultures of normal kidney tissue. Cytogenet Cell Genet 1990;53:123–125.

105 Elfving P, Aman P, Mandahl N, Lundgren R, Mitelman F: Trisomy 7 in nonneoplastic epithelial kidney cells. Cytogenet Cell Genet 1995;69:90–96.

106 Bugert P, Gaul C, Weber K, Herbers J, Akhtar M, Ljungberg B, Kovacs G: Specific genetic changes of diagnostic importance in chromophobe renal cell carcinomas. Lab Invest 1997;76:203–208.

107 Moch H, Presti JC, Sauter G, Buchholz N, Jordan P, Mihatsch MJ, Waldman FM: Genetic aberrations deteced by comparative genomic hybridization are associated with clinical outcome in renal cell carcinoma. Cancer Res 1996;56:27–30.

Eva van den Berg, PhD, Department of Medical Genetics, University of Groningen,
Antonius Deusinglaan 4, NL–9713 AW Groningen (The Netherlands)
Tel. +31 50 3632938, Fax +31 50 3632457, E-Mail E.van.den.Berg-de.Ruiter@med.rug.nl

Hino O (ed): Kidney Cancer. Recent Results of Basic and Clinical Research.
Contrib Nephrol. Basel, Karger, 1999, vol 128, pp 62–74

Wilms' Tumor and the *WT1* Gene

Jun-ichi Hata

Department of Pathology, Keio University School of Medicine, Tokyo, Japan

Introduction

Wilms' tumor or nephroblastoma is a childhood kidney tumor that is thought to arise from cells of the metanephric blastema, a fetal kidney structure. The occurrence of both sporadic and hereditary forms, along with various congenital abnormalities of Wilms' tumor, suggests that the tumors develop when a predisposing germ line mutation is accompanied by a second mutation. The existence of both gross chromosomal abnormalities has led to the genetic characterization of a number of loci involved in the development of Wilms' tumor. A tumor-suppressor gene for Wilms' tumor, *WT1*, has recently been isolated from the distal 11p13 region. The product of this gene is a transcription factor with four zinc fingers. Because expression of *WT1* is limited to the developing glomeruli of the kidneys and the genital ridge, it is thought to have a functional role in renal and gonadal organogenesis. Thus dysfunction of *WT1* causes loss of normal regulation of proliferation and leads to tumor formation and occurrence of Wilms' tumor anomaly complexes. In this paper, recent topics related to the *WT1* gene and Wilms' tumor are discussed.

Wilms' Tumor

Wilms' tumor is derived from the metanephric blastema. During human nephrogenesis, the metanephric blastema differentiates into glomeruli and proximal and distal tubules with strong induction by the ureteric buds before 30 weeks of gestation, and tumorigenesis may occur during this process of differentiation into glomeruli and renal tubules. The tumor tissue, therefore, mimics the developing renal cortex [1]. Tumor blastema can differentiate into

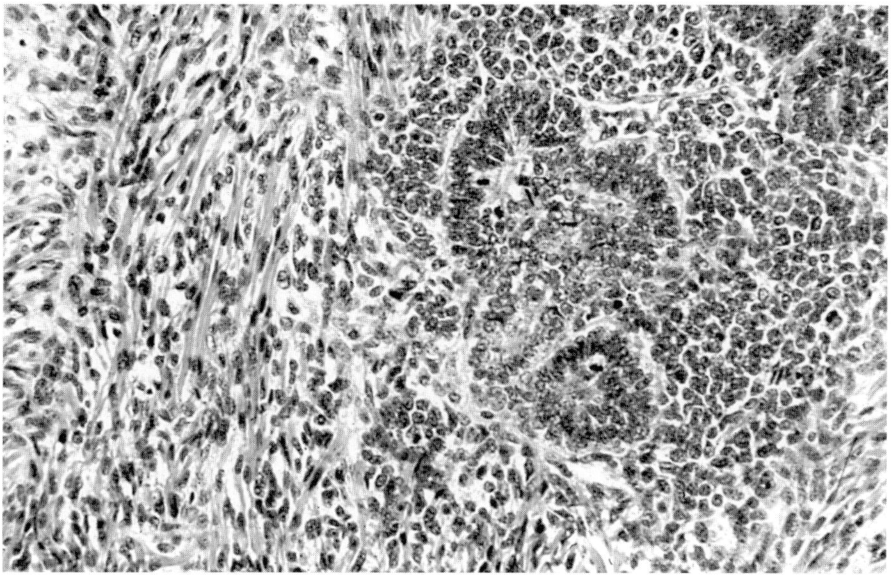

Fig. 1. Histology of nephroblastic Wilms' tumor. Note immature blastemal, epithelial and striated muscle components. HE.

epithelial cells and into mesenchymal cells, such as striated muscle cells, smooth muscle cells and cartilagenous tissue. Thus the histological features of Wilms' tumors are composed of epithelial and mesenchymal components as well as immature blastemal cells. Such tumors are also termed 'classical' or 'nephroblastic' Wilms' tumors (fig. 1, 2).

A variety of congenital malformations occur in association with Wilms' tumor, and they are closely related to the pattern of chromosomal abnormalities [2]. Aniridia and hypospadia are abnormalities associated with deletions at 11p13 [3, 4]. Wilms' tumor anomaly complex syndrome, such as Wilms' tumor-anidiria-genitourinary-anomaly syndrome which consists of aniridia, genitourinary malformations, mental retardation and Denys-Drash syndrome, is characterized by progressive renal failure, Wilms' tumor and abnormal sex differentiation due to XY gonadal dysgenesis, and is also associated with deletion of 11p13 [5]. Hemihypertrophy and Beckwith-Wiedemann syndrome are Wilms' tumor anomaly complex syndromes associated with abnormalities at 11p15 [6]. Macroglossia, hemihypertrophy, umbilical hernia, and adrenal gland cytomegaly are also observed in this syndrome [7–9]. Approximately 10% of patients with this syndrome also have malignant embryonic tumors such as hepatoblastomas and Wilms' tumors [10–14].

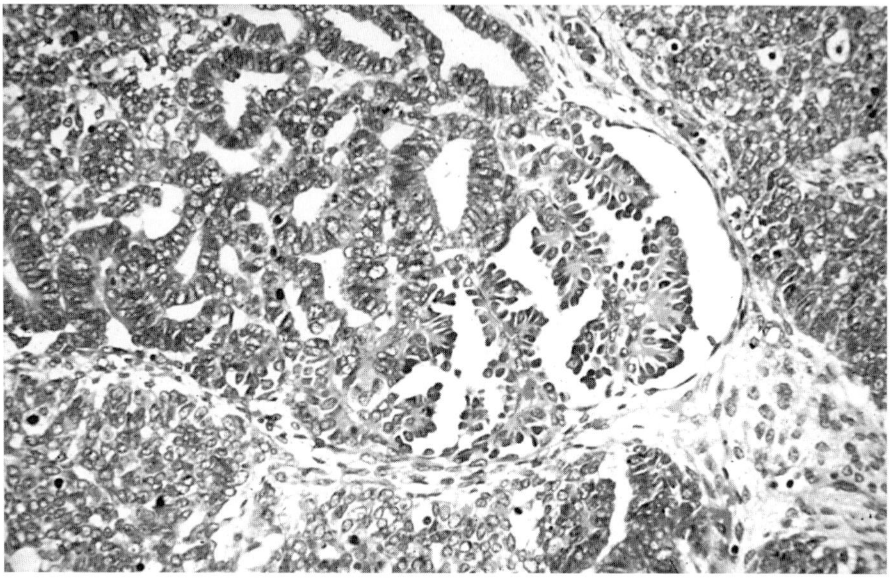

Fig. 2. Histology of nephroblastic Wilms' tumor. Tumor tissue mimics glomerular structure. HE.

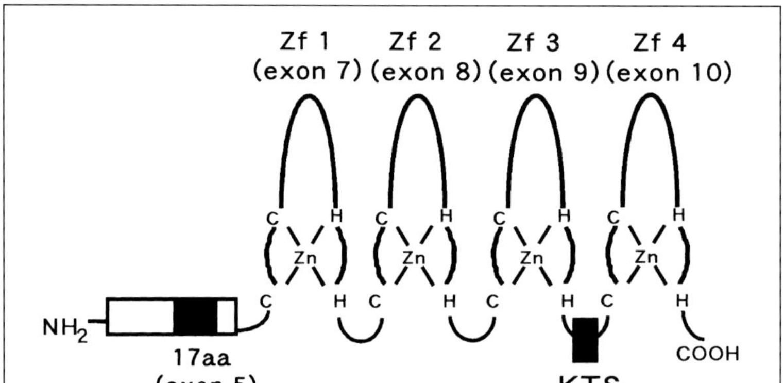

Fig. 3. Structure of *WT1* gene. Zf = Zinc finger domain; KTS = lysine, threonine, serine. Black boxes indicate alternative splice sites.

a 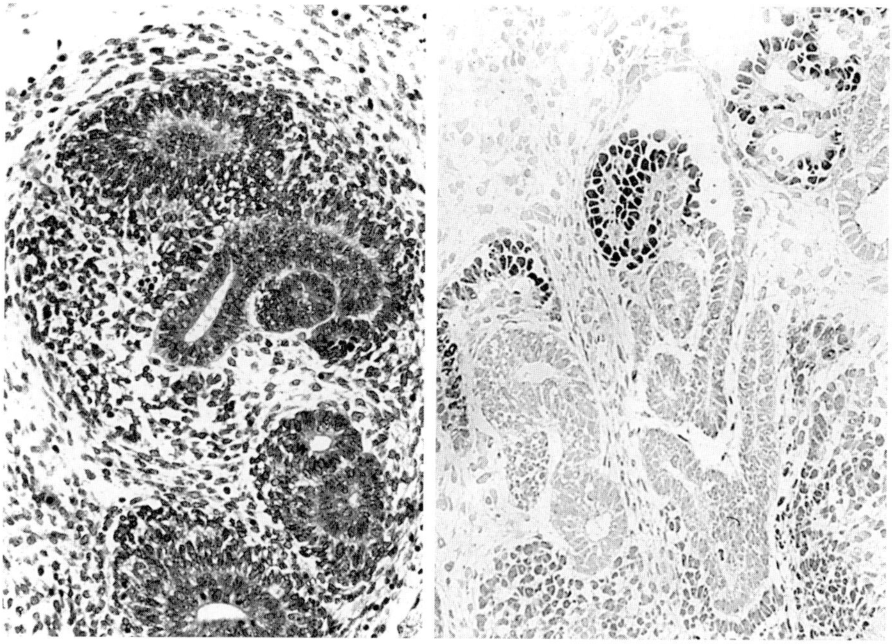 b

Fig. 4. Developing human renal cortex (4th gestational week). *a* HE. *b WT1* immunostaining. Developing podocytes are positive for *WT1* protein.

Structure and Functions of the *WT1* Gene

In 1990, the *WT1* tumor-suppressor gene, which is responsible for the development of Wilms' tumor, was cloned from the distal part of 11p13 [15,16]. The *WT1* gene contains 10 exons and encodes a transcription factor containing four Cys_2-His_2 zinc fingers and a proline/glutamine-rich amino terminus (fig. 3). These zinc finger domains bind a specific DNA sequence (-GCGGGGGCG-) [17]. WT1 proteins have been shown to regulate the expression of early growth response factor-1, insulin-like growth factor-2 (IGF-2), IGF-2 receptor, platelet-derived growth factor-A and Pax-2 at the transcriptional level [18–21]. There are four WT1 protein isoforms resulting from two alternative splicing sites. The first site involves the presence or absence of 17 amino acids encoded by exon 5, while the second involves inclusion or exclusion of three amino acids, lysine, threonine and serine (KTS), between the third and fourth zinc finger domains. *WT1* is only expressed in a limited range of tissues such as the fetal kidneys, especially in developing glomerular podocytes (fig. 4) [22–24]. It is also stage-specifically expressed in the genital ridge (fig. 5),

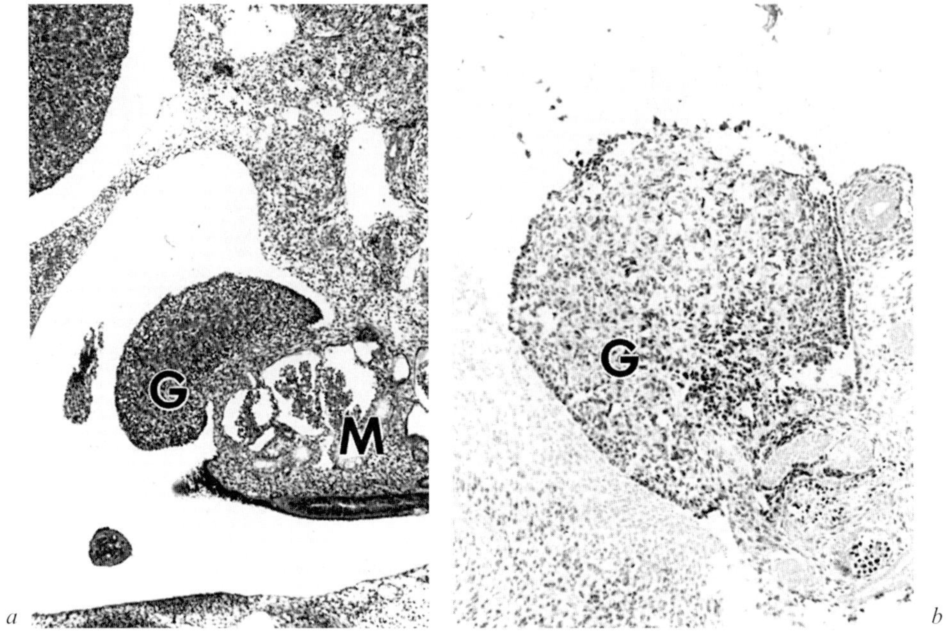

Fig. 5. Human genital ridges (4th gestational week). *a* HE. G = Genital ridge; M = mesonephros. *b WT1* immunostaining. Genital ridge is positive for *WT1* protein.

which is the anlage of the stromal cells of the testes and ovaries, and in mesothelial cells, the spleen and leukemic cells [25, 26]. Targeted mutation of *WT1* led to apoptosis in the metanephric blastemal cells of fetuses and failure of the kidney to develop [23]. It also led to atrophy of the genital ridge, the anlage of gonadal stromal cells. Of these stromal cells, the Sertoli cells observed in seminiferous tubuli of fetal and adult testes are believed to be essential for the development of male internal and external sex organs through the activation of the sex-determining gene *SRY* on the Y chromosome. These findings suggested that *WT1* plays an important role in the development of kidneys and male genital organs, and sex differentiation.

There are some Wilms' tumor anomaly complexes such as Denys-Drash syndrome consisting of Wilms' tumor, congenital nephropathy caused by diffuse mesangeal sclerosis, and XY gonadal dysgenesis [27]. Patients with Denys-Drash syndrome almost always carry point mutation in the zinc finger regions of *WT1* [28]. Based upon these findings, *WT1* is thought to play a crucial role in the development of the kidney and male sex organs. Accordingly, dysfunction of the gene leads to both Wilms' tumor development and urogenital abnormalities.

WT1 Abnormalities and Wilms' Tumor Development

The frequency of *WT1* mutations in sporadic Wilms' tumor is said to be approximately 15% [29, 30]. We detected 5 cases with genomic deletion in 60 Wilms' tumor cases by Southern blot analysis [31]. In addition, we detected another 6 cases of *WT1* gene mutation by direct sequencing of PCR products (unpubl. data). The range of the mutations extended to almost all exons including point mutations associated with nonsense mutations in exons 8 and 9, which are the zinc finger domains, and insertion of 46 basepairs resulting in loss of the stop codon (unpubl. data) [32, 33]. These mutations were more diverse than those associated with Wilms' tumor anomaly complexes, as described later. However, the low frequency of *WT1* mutations in sporadic Wilms' tumor suggests that other genes located in the 11p15 region, such as H19 and IGF2, may also play a role in tumor development [34–38].

WT1 Gene Abnormalities in Wilms' Tumor Anomaly Complex Syndromes

In contrast to sporadic Wilms' tumor, the *WT1* gene has been shown to be responsible for Denys-Drash syndrome [39]. This syndrome is characterized by early onset and progressive renal failure due to diffuse mesangial sclerosis, Wilms' tumors and XY gonadal dysgenesis (female external genitalia and streak gonads despite a 46,XY karyotype). These genital abnormalities are thought to be due to dysfunction of *WT1* gene expressed in the stromal cell of the genital ridge. *WT1* gene dysfunction may lead to maldeveloped Sertoli cells resulting in a functional deficiency in the Mullerian duct inhibitory factor, which plays a crucial role in development of male sex organs and in incomplete masculinization (XY female). Pelletier et al. [40] postulated that when a point mutation in the zinc finger domain of *WT1* occurred in one allele at the somatic cell (germ line) level, it caused nephropathy and intersex abnormalities by dominant negative effects, and that when it occurred in both alleles in the kidney, it caused Wilms' tumor and induced the same syndrome. Almost all reported cases of Denys-Drash syndrome had point mutations within zinc finger regions [41].

We identified point mutations in the zinc finger regions in all 11 cases clinically diagnosed as Denys-Drash syndrome (table 1). Analysis of the *WT1* gene from 11 patients that we examined was carried out by direct sequencing of PCR products of exons 7–10 which encode zinc finger domains. Point mutations of the *WT1* gene involving one allele were recognized in all patients. Four of the mutations were in exons and five were in introns (table 2). Because

Table 1. Clinical diagnosis of Drash syndrome

Case No.	Age years	Nephropathy (age at dialysis)	Histology	Karyotype external/internal genitalia	Tumor
E-1	1	RF (1 year)	FGS	46,XX normal	Wilms' tumor
E-2	2	RF (2 years)	FGS	46,XY female/streak gonads	No
E-3	5	RF (1 month)		46,XX normal	Wilms' tumor
E-4	7	RF (1 year)	DMS	46,XY female	No
I-1[a]	18	NS	FGS	46,XY female/streak gonads	No
I-2[a]	18	NS	FGS	46,XY female/streak gonads	No
I-3[a]	19	RF (16 years)	FGS	46,XY female/streak gonads	No
I-4	3	Proteinuria		46,XY female	No
I-5	26	RF (23 years)	FGS	46,XY female/streak gonads	No
I-6	19	RF (12 years)	FGSG	46,XY female	No
I-7	15	RF (8 years)		46,XY female	No

E = Exonic mutation cases; I = intronic mutation cases; NS = nephrotic syndrome; RF = renal failure.

[a] Cases I-1 and 2 are identical twins.

the intron mutations were suspected to lead to abnormal splicing, we used a *WT1* minigene for confirmation. Four representative minigene inserts, one normal and three intron mutations detected in the patients, were made and inserted into an expression vector. COS-7 cells were transfected with these constructs and the transcripts were then analyzed by RT-PCR. Interestingly, only one amplified product that corresponded to the transcript without nine nucleotides was obtained from the mutant minigenes, whereas two products (with or without nine bases) were obtained from the normal constructs (fig. 6). The intron mutations affecting alternative splicing between exons 9 and 10 prevent production of the transcripts with nine nucleotides. This minigene

Table 2. *WT1* mutations in Drash syndrome

Case No.	*WT1* mutation		
	exon/intron	DNA	amino acid
E-1	exon 8 (1064)	CAGTATGAC ↑ CAGTGTGAC	^{355}Thr←^{355}Cys
E-2	exon 9 (1154)	CAGCGTAAA ↑ CAGTGTAAA	^{385}Arg←^{385}Cys
E-3	exon 8 (1097)	TTTCATTCA ↑ TTTCGTTCA	^{366}His←^{366}Arg
E-4	exon 7 (1025)	CAGAGGCAC ↑ CAGATGCAC	^{342}Arg←^{342}Met
I-1, 2, 3	intron 9 (+4)	gtgtg ↑ gtgcg	Disruption of alternative splicing
I-4	intron 9 (+5)	gtgct ↑ gtgcg	Disruption of alternative splicing
I-5, 7	intron 9 (+2)	gcgcg ↑ gtgcg	Disruption of alternative splicing
I-6	intron 9 (+5)	gtgca ↑ gtgcg	Disruption of alternative splicing

assay provided in vitro confirmation that all of these mutations affect post-transcriptional processing of RNA, preventing production of the splicing variant with 9 bases. This suggested that imbalance of the alternative splicing isoforms of *WT1* is involved in the pathogenesis of the symptoms in these patients.

When we carefully reexamined the clinical features of patients with intronic mutations, these were highly consistent with those of Frasier syndrome, proposed by Moorthy et al. [42] to be related to, but distinct from Denys-Drash syndrome. The onset of nephropathy is very early in Denys-Drash syndrome, usually in the first year of life, progressing to end-stage renal failure by 3 years

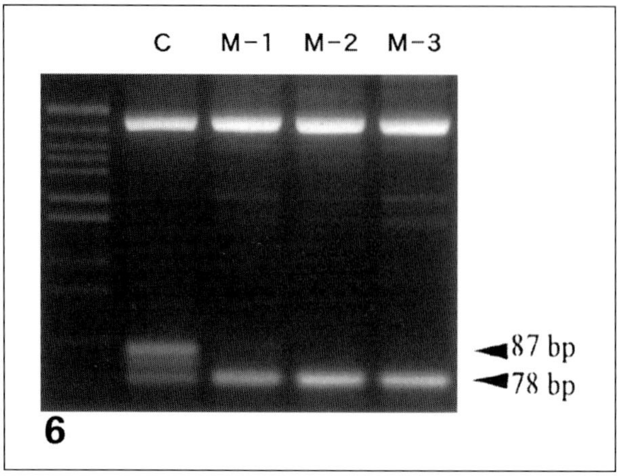

Fig. 6. RT-PCR products from COS-7 cells transfected with *WT1* minigenes. The 87-bp size band corresponding to product containing +KTS was detected only in the normal minigene. M-1, 2, 3 = Products from mutated *WT1* constructs; C = product from normal *WT1* construct; M-1 = intron +4c to t(I-1, 2, 3); M-2 = +5g to t(I-4); M-3 = t to c(I-5). From Kikuchi et al. [41].

of age. In Frasier syndrome, renal histology reveals features of focal glomerular sclerosis. The onset of nephropathy is at 4 years or older and the clinical course is slowly progressive, requiring at least 2 years to reach end-stage renal failure. On the other hand, patients with intronic mutations had uniform genital systems. Their external genitalia were female despite a 46,XY karyotype. None of our patients or those reported to have intron 9 splicing donor site mutations developed Wilms' tumor. This is in contrast to an incidence of Wilms' tumor of 55% among patients with Denys-Drash syndrome. This absence of Wilms' tumor development is one of the major criteria for Frasier syndrome. In our study, all of the patients with intronic mutations were 46,XY female, although the same mutations can be theoretically expected to occur in cases with a 46,XX karyotype as well. This is probably because in 46,XX karyotypic patients the diagnosis of Denys-Drash (or Frasier) syndrome is very often difficult as the malformations observed in the external genitalia are usually mild in these cases.

In summary, patients with mutations of the *WT1* gene intron 9 splicing donor site showed characteristics which were entirely consistent with Frasier syndrome. In terms of pathogenesis, both Denys-Drash syndrome and Frasier syndrome are caused by specific mutations of the same gene, *WT1*. If the mutations occur in particular exon regions, the outcome is Denys-Drash syn-

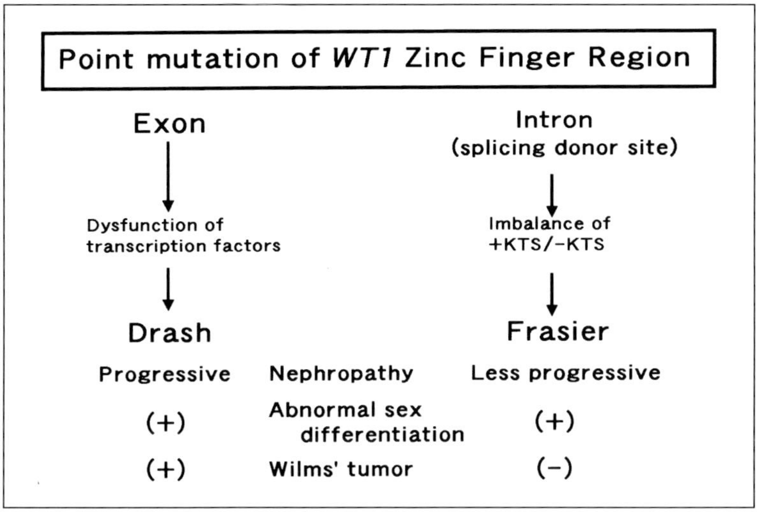

Fig. 7. Molecular pathogenesis of Drash and Frasier syndrome.

drome, while mutations in the splicing donor site of intron 9 cause a series of common abnormalities defined as Frasier syndrome (fig. 7). These findings also suggest a molecular mechanism for the effect of splicing donor site mutations of *WT1* intron 9. In patients with Denys-Drash syndrome specific alterations of the *WT1* gene produce dominant-negative proteins, resulting in inactivation of the product from the normal allele. In contrast, only normal products are present in patients with intron mutations. A normal quantity of *WT1* isoforms without KTS is produced, but the quantity of isoforms with KTS is insufficient due to the intron mutations. Consequently, an imbalance in the ratio of +KTS/ –KTS isoforms, presumably half normal versus normal, is thought to produce the characteristic clinical picture known as Frasier syndrome [41, 43].

A recent study of the subnuclear localization of these *WT1* isoforms revealed different localization. The +KTS *WT1* proteins are localized mainly with splicing factors and appear to be involved in post-transcriptional RNA processing. While –KTS forms are found in the transcriptional factor domains and are thus likely to bind DNA [44]. Therefore, it is possible that *WT1* proteins produced by alternative splicing of exon 9 have different functions in the development of different organs and in tumorigenesis, and that this difference might explain the characteristic features of Frasier syndrome. Since the –KTS isoforms usually bind to genes related to growth with higher affinity, loss of the functions of these isoforms may be more closely related to the development of Wilms' tumor. Both +KTS and –KTS may be necessary for renal organogenesis, and +KTS isoforms appear to play a key role in the development of gonadal tissues. Confirmation of this hypothesis requires further study of the precise functions of both *WT1* alternative splicing products, especially in developing kidneys and gonads. At the same time, identification of *WT1* mutations is also useful in predicting the outcome of intractable nephropathy and the development of Wilms' tumor.

References

1 Beckwith JB, Kiviat NB, Bonadio JF: Nephrogenic rests, nephroblastomatosis, and the pathogenesis of Wilms' tumor. Pediatr Pathol 1990;10:1–36.

2 Green DM, Breslow NE, Beckwith JB, Norkool P: Screening of children with hemihypertrophy, aniridia, and Beckwith-Wiedemann syndrome in patients with Wilms tumor: A report from the National Wilms Tumor Study. Med Pediatr Oncol 1993;21:188–192.

3 Slater RM, Mannens MM: Cytogenetics and molecular genetics of Wilms' tumor of childhood. Cancer Genet Cytogenet 1992;61:111–121.

4 Newsham I, Cavenee W: Tumors and developmental anomalies associated with Wilms' tumor. Med Pediatr Oncol 1993;21:199–204.

5 Craft AW, Parker L, Stiller C, Cole M: Screening for Wilms' tumour in patients with aniridia, Beckwith syndrome, or hemihypertrophy. Med Pediatr Oncol 1995;24:231–234.

6 Feinberg AP: Multiple genetic abnormalities of 11p15 in Wilms' tumor. Med Pediatr Oncol 1996; 27:484–489.

7 Eaton AP, Maurer WF: The Beckwith-Wiedemann syndrome. Am J Dis Child 1971;122:520–525.

8 Elliott M, Maher ER: Beckwith-Wiedemann syndrome. J Med Genet 1994;31:560–564.

9 Engstrom W, Lindham S, Schofield P: Wiedemann-Beckwith syndrome. Eur J Pediatr 1988;147: 450–457.

10 Sotelo-Avila C, Gooch WMD: Neoplasms associated with the Beckwith-Wiedemann syndrome. Perspect Pediatr Pathol 1976;3:255–272.

11 Hecht F, Sandberg AA: Wiedemann-Beckwith syndrome: Cancer predisposition and chromosome 11. Cancer Genet Cytogenet 1986;23:159–161.

12 Reik W, Brown KW, Schneid H, Le Bouc Y, Bickmore W, Maher ER: Imprinting mutations in the Beckwith-Wiedemann syndrome suggested by altered imprinting pattern in the IGF2-H19 domain. Hum Mol Genet 1995;4:2379–2385.

13 Schneid H, Vazquez MP, Vacher C, Gourmelen M, Cabrol S, Le Bouc Y: The Beckwith-Wiedemann syndrome phenotype and the risk of cancer. Med Pediatr Oncol 1997;28:411–415.

14 Choyke PL, Siegel MJ, Craft AW, Green DM, DeBaun MR: Screening for Wilms tumor in children with Beckwith-Wiedemann syndrome or idiopathic hemihypertrophy. Med Pediatr Oncol 1999;32: 196–200.

15 Call K, Glase T, Ito CY, Buckler AJ, Pelletier J, Harber DA, Rose EA, Kral A, Yeger H, Lewis WH, Gones C, Houseman DE: Isolation and characterization of a zinc finger polypeptide gene at the human chromosome 11 Wilms' tumor locus. Cell 1990;60:509–520.

16 Gessler M, Poustha A, Cavenee W, Neve RL, Orkin S, Bruns GAP: Homozygous deletion of Wilms' tumors of a zinc-finger gene identified by chromosome jumping. Nature 1990;343:774–778.

17 Rauscher FJ III, Morris JF, Tournay OE, Cook DM, Curran T: Binding of the Wilms' tumor locus zinc finger protein to the EGR-1 consensus sequence. Science 1990;250:1259–1262.

18 Drummond IA, Madden SL, Rohwer-Nutter P, Bell GI, Sukhatme VP, Rauscher FJ III: Repression of the insulin-like growth factor II gene by the Wilms tumor suppressor *WT1*. Science 1992;257: 674–678.

19 Wang ZY, Qiu QQ, Enger KT, Deuel TF: A second transcriptionally active DNA-binding site for the Wilms tumor gene product, *WT1*. Proc Natl Acad Sci USA 1993;90:8896–900.

20 Werner H, Rauscher Fr, Sukhatme VP, Drummond IA, Roberts CJ, LeRoith D: Transcriptional repression of the insulin-like growth factor I receptor (IGF-I-R) gene by the tumor suppressor *WT1* involves binding to sequences both upstream and downstream of the IGF-I-R gene transcription start site. J Biol Chem 1994;269:12577–12582.
21 Sells SF, Muthukumar S, Sukhatme VP, Crist SA, Rangnekar VM: The zinc finger transcription factor EGR-1 impedes interleukin-1-inducible tumor growth arrest. Mol Cell Biol 1995;15:682–692.
22 Pritchard-Jones K, Flemming S, Davidson D, Bickmore W, Porteous D, Gosden C, Bard J, Buckler A, Pelletier J, Housman D, Heyningen V, Hastie N: The candidate Wilms' tumor gene is involved in genitourinary development. Nature 1990;346:194–197.
23 Keridberg J, Sariola H, Loring J, Maeda M, Pelletier J, Housman D, Jaenisch R: *WT1* required for early kidney development. Cell 1993;74:679–691.
24 Kritz W, Grets N, Lemley K: Progression of glomerular dieases: Is the podocyte the culprit? Kidney Int 1998;54:687–697.
25 van Heyningen V, Bickmore WA, Seawright A, Fletcher JM, Maule J, Fekete G, Gessler M, Bruns GA: Role for the Wilms tumor gene in genital development? Proc Natl Acad Sci USA 1990;87: 5383–5386.
26 Walker C, Rutten F, Yuan X, Pass H, Mew DM, Everitt J: Wilms' tumor suppressor gene expression in rat and human mesothelioma. Cancer Res 1994;54:3101–3106.
27 Drash A, Sherman F, Hartman WH, Blizzard RM: A syndrome of peudohermaphroditism, nephritis, Wilms' tumor, hypertension and degenerative renal disease. J Pediatr 1970;76:585.
28 Coppes MJ, Huff V, Pelletier J: Denys-Drash syndrome: Relating a clinical disorder to genetic alterations in the tumor suppressor gene *WT1*. J Pediatr 1993;123:673–678.
29 Varanasi R, Bardeesy N, Ghahremani M, Petruzzi MJ, Nowak N, Adam MA, Grundy P: Fine structure analysis of the *WT1* gene in sporadic Wilms tumors. Proc Natl Acad Sci USA 1994;91: 3554–3558.
30 Gessler M, Konig A, Arden K, Grundy P, Orkin S, Sallan S, Peters C, Ruyle S: Infrequent mutation of the *WT1* gene in 77 Wilms' tumors. Hum Mutat 1994;3:212–222.
31 Kikuchi H, Akasaka Y, Nagai T, Kato S, Hata J: Genomic changes in WT-gene *(WT1)* in Wilms' tumors and their correlation with histology. Am J Pathol 1992;140:781–784.
32 Akasaka Y, Kikuchi H, Nagai T, Hiraoka N, Kato S, Hata J: A point mutation found in the *WT1* gene in a sporadic Wilms' tumor without genitourinary abnormalities is identical with the most frequent point mutation in Denys-Drash syndrome. FEBS Lett 1993;317:39–43.
33 Huff V: Genotype/phenotype correlations in Wilms' tumor. Med Pediatr Oncol 1996;27:408–414.
34 Kikuchi H, Akasaka Y, Kurosawa Y, Yoneyama H, Kato S, Hata J: A critical mutation in both *WT1* alleles is not sufficient to cause Wilms' tumor. FEBS Lett 1995;360:16–18.
35 Taniguchi T, Sullivan MJ, Ogawa O, Reeve AE: Epigenetic changes encompassing the IGF2/H19 locus associated with relaxation of IGF2 imprinting and silencing of H19 in Wilms tumor. Proc Natl Acad Sci USA 1995;92:2159–2163.
36 Moulton T, Chung WY, Yuan L: Genomic imprinting and Wilms' tumor. Med Pediatr Oncol 1996; 27:476–483.
37 Reeve AE: Role of genomic imprinting in Wilms' tumour and overgrowth disorders. Med Pediatr Oncol 1996;27:470–475.
38 Cui H, Hedborg F, He L, Nordenskjold A, Sandstedt B, Pfeifer-Ohlsson S, Ohlsson R: Inactivation of H19, an imprinted and putative tumor repressor gene, is a preneoplastic event during Wilms' tumorigenesis. Cancer Res 1997;57:4469–4473.
39 Little M, Holmes G, Bickmore W, van Heyningen V, Hastie N, Wainwright B: DNA binding capacity of the *WT1* protein is abolished by Denys-Drash syndrome *WT1* point mutations. Hum Mol Genet 1995;4:351–358.
40 Pelletier J, Bruening W, Kashtan CE, Mauer SM, Manivel JC, Striegel JE, Bardeesy N, Silberman B, Haber DA, Housman D: Germ line mutations in the Wilms' tumor suppressor genes are associated with abnormal urogenital development in Dynes-Drash syndrome. Cell 1991;67:437–447.
41 Kikuchi H, Takata A, Hata J: Do intronic mutations affecting splicing of *WT1* exon 9 cause Frasier syndrome? J Med Genet 1998;35:45–48.

42 Moorthy A, Chesney R, Lubinsky M: Chronic renal failure and XY gonadal dysgenesis: 'Frasier syndrome' – A commentary on reported cases. Am J Med Genet 1987(suppl 3):297–302.
43 Babaux S, Nitauder P, Gulber M-C, Nitauder P, Gulber M-C, Grunfeld J-P, Jaubert F, Kutenn F, Fekete CN, Therville N, Tahibaud E, Fellous M, McElreavy K: Donor splice-site mutations in *WT1* are responsible for Frasier syntrome. Nat Genet 1997;17:467–469.
44 Larsson SH, Charlieu J, Miyagawa K, Engelkamp D, Rassoulzadegen M, Ross A, Cuzin F, van Haynigen V, Hastie ND: Subnuclear localization of *WT1* in splicing or transcription factor domains is regulated by alternative splicing. Cell 1995;81:391–401.

Jun-ichi Hata, MD, PhD, Department of Pathology, Keio University School of Medicine,
35 Shinanomachi, Shinjuku-ku, Tokyo 160-8582 (Japan)
Tel. +81 3 5363 3762, Fax +81 3 3353 3290, E-Mail jhata@med.keio.ac.jp

Hino O (ed): Kidney Cancer. Recent Results of Basic and Clinical Research.
Contrib Nephrol. Basel, Karger, 1999, vol 128, pp 75–81

Gene-Modified Immunotherapy for Renal Cell Carcinoma

Koji Kawai[a], *Kenzaburo Tani*[b], *Shigetaka Asano*[b], *Hideyuki Akaza*[a]

[a] Department of Urology, Institute of Clinical Medicine, University of Tsukuba, Tsukuba City, and
[b] Department of Hematology/Oncology, Institute of Medical Science, University of Tokyo, Japan

Introduction

Treatment results for metastatic renal carcinoma (RCC) remain poor largely due to the chemotherapy-resistant nature of this cancer. The relatively high response rate to various types of immunomodulatory agents suggests that RCC is an immunogeneic cancer similar to melanoma. With recent advances in molecular biology, a number of preclinical studies and clinical protocols using gene modification have been conducted to overcome the limitations of systemic therapy for cancer [1, 2]. In RCC, gene-modified immunotherapy is considered to be a promising treatment modality for patients with metastasis. We briefly reviewed the current approaches to tumor-specific immunotherapy using gene modification.

Limitations of Conventional Immunotherapy for Metastatic RCC

There is no effective systemic therapy for metastatic RCC. Although various cytokine therapies using interferons or interleukin (IL)-2 produced favorable clinical responses in some patients, the overall response rate based on cumulative data has been reported to range from 12 to 20% [3]. Another approach which has been investigated in RCC is adoptive immunotherapy using ex vivo expanded immune cells. Two types of activated cells have been employed in metastatic RCC patients: lymphokine activated killer (LAK) cells derived from peripheral blood lymphocytes, and tumor-infiltrating lymphocytes (TILs) isolated from surgically resected cancer tissue. Although promising results were shown in some clinical studies [4], adoptive immunotherapies with LAK and bulk TIL have not yet been proven beneficial in the treatment of metastatic RCC [5]. Several reasons for the limited efficacy were proposed, i.e., a heterogeneous population of infused effector cells; poor localization of the transferred effector cells to tumor sites, and suboptimal activity of the effector cells at the local tumor sites.

Prospectives of Tumor-Specific Immunotherapy for RCC

Since the establishment of methods to isolate genes encoding tumor antigen recognized by cytotoxic T lymphocyte (CTL), numerous tumor-associated antigens (TAAs) were identified in melanoma and various types of cancer [6]. In contrast to natural killer cells or LAK cells, CTL is known to have high and specific cytotoxic activity against cancer cells recognizing TAAs in a major histocompatibility complex (MHC)-restricted manner. CTL is considered to play a significant role in tumor regression in melanoma and RCC patients receiving high-dose IL-2 therapy or TIL therapy [7, 8]. This finding suggests that RCC, like melanoma, expresses specific antigens that can be recognized by the CTL. Recently, the expression of TAAs such as RAGE-1, mutated HLA-A2 protein or other melanoma-associated antigens were observed in RCC specimens or RCC cell lines [9–11]. However, only limited data are available regarding whether CTL can recognize those putative TAAs in RCC. Thus, until more common TAAs have been identified in RCC, each individual's tumor is the only source of TAAs for generating a tumor-specific immune reaction against RCC. One possible approach is adoptive cell therapy using ex vivo selectively expanded CTLs. Recently, several investigators have reported efficient culture methods to generate RCC-specific CTL [12, 13]. Another approach is in vivo vaccination using gene-modified tumor cells to enhance host immunity against the tumor.

Preclinical Studies in Gene-Modified Immunotherapy

There have been various approaches in cancer gene therapy such as tumor-suppressor gene, pro-drug strategy using suicide gene, and gene-modified immunotherapy. Among them, gene-modified tumor vaccine strategies have been most intensively studied in both preclinical and clinical studies [1, 14]. In animal models, a number of cytokine genes were found to reduce the tumorigenicity of

Table 1. Preclinical studies in gene-modified immunotherapy [15–20]

Tumor	Cytokines	Protection against rechallenge	Tumor regression	Proposed mechanism or major effector cell
CT26 (colon)	IL-2	+	ND	CTL activity
WP-4 (sarcoma)	TNF	+	ND	CD4+ or CD8+ T cell
Renca (renal cell)	IL-4	+	+	CD8+ T cell
Lewis (lung)	IL-6	+	+	CTL activity
J558 (plasmacytoma)	IL-7	+	ND	CD4+ T cell and macrophage
B16 (melanoma)	GM-CSF	+	+	CD4+ or CD8+ T cell

transduced cancer cells by local inflammatory or immune responses. In a model subset, more importantly, inoculation of cytokine-engineered cells induces tumor-specific immune responses as defined by protecting the animal from rechallenge with parental tumor cells, or by regression of established parental tumors (table 1) [15–20]. Although several cellular and humoral mechanisms are considered to be involved in tumor rejection, many investigators suggested a significant role of T-cell-mediated tumor immunity. In some studies, CTL activity against parental tumor cells was demonstrated in splenocytes of animals injected with cytosine-expressing tumor. Although several kinds of cytokines showed the activity, granulocyte-macrophage colony-stimulating factor (GM-CSF) is considered to be a promising candidate for augmenting immunity [20]. GM-CSF has shown the most potent activity by comparing the relative activity of different gene products in a single tumor model. In addition, Dranoff et al. [20] demonstrated the efficacy of GM-CSF-transduced vaccines by comparing the activity of transduced tumor cells to that of nontransduced cells in animal models of colon cancer, prostate cancer and RCC [20]. Since CD4 and CD8 before and after GM-CSF vaccination abrogated the anti-tumor activity, both subsets of T cells were critical for systemic immunity of GM-CSF-transduced vaccine. Figure 1 illustrates a proposed mechanism involved in systemic immunity induced by GM-CSF-transduced vaccination. The action of GM-CSF involves the local spread of cytokines at high concentrations which activated the function of antigen-presenting cells (APCs) including macrophages and dendritic cells. The dendritic cell is known to be the most potent APC for helper T cells. Both CD4+ and CD8+ T cells are activated which results in destruction of tumor cells at metastatic sites upon T-cell recognition of TAAs.

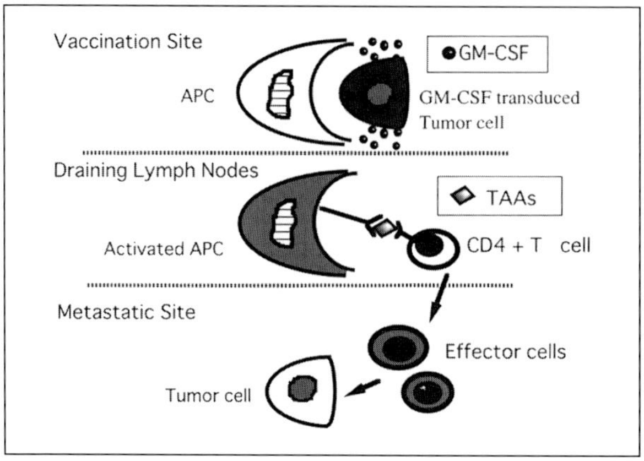

Fig. 1. Proposed mechanism in systemic immunity in GM-CSF-transduced tumor vaccination.

Table 2. Results of a phase-I study of an autologous GM-CSF gene-transduced tumor vaccine for RCC patients

	GM-CSF –	GM-CSF +
Cell dose		
Level 1, 4×10^6	3	4
Level 2, 4×10^7	4	3
Level 3, 4×10^8	2	–
GM-CSF secretion, ng/10^6 cell/24 h	0–19	42–149
DTH response to RCC cell	5/9	4/7
Tumor response		
Level 1	0/3	0/4
Level 2	0/4	1/3
Level 3	0/2	–

Results of Phase-I Study of an Autologous GM-CSF Gene-Transduced Tumor Vaccine for RCC Patients and Other Clinical Studies of Gene-Modifed Immunotherapy for RCC

The first ex vivo gene therapy trial for the treatment of metastatic RCC was conducted at Johns Hopkins Oncology Center using GM-CSF gene-transduced tumor vaccines (table 2) [21]. In this double-blinded trial, patients were randomized to treatment with escalating doses of autologous tumor vaccine with or

Table 3. Current gene therapy approaches for RCC

Gene	Gene transfection	Target	Delivery vehicle	Institute
TNF	Ex vivo	Autologous RCC cell	Retrovirus	NIH
IL-2	Ex vivo	Autologous RCC cell	Retrovirus	NIH
IL-2	Ex vivo	Allogeneic RCC cell (HLA-matched)	Retrovirus	MSKCC
IL-4	Ex vivo	Autologous fibroblast (with untransduced RCC cell)	Retrovirus	University of Pittsburg
GM-CSF	Ex vivo	Autologous RCC cell	Retrovirus	Johns Hopkins Oncology Center/Institute of Medical Science, University of Tokyo
HLA-B7/β_2-microglobulin	Ex vivo	Autologous RCC cell	Lipid	Providence Medical Center
HLA-B7/β_2-microglobulin	In vivo	Direct intratumoral injection	Lipid	Phase II study
HLA-B7	In vivo	Direct intratumoral injection	Lipid	UCLA Medical Center
IL-2	In vivo	Direct intratumoral injection	Lipid	UCLA Medical Center
B7.1 (CD80)	Ex vivo	Autologous RCC cell	Adenovirus	University of Southern California

without ex vivo GM-CSF gene transfer. Autologous tumor cells were harvested from primary tumors and transfected with a retroviral vector carrying the GM-CSF gene. The transduced and untransduced tumor cells were then irradiated and administered to the patients. Through dose escalation, no dose-limiting side effects were observed in 16 patients. One partial response was observed in a patient with multiple lung metastases treated with GM-CSF gene-transduced vaccine. During the trial, several types of immune parameters including delayed-type hypersensitivity (DTH) against autologous irradiated RCC cells were monitored. The patient with partial response displayed the largest DTH conversion in this trial. No replication-competent retrovirus was detected in vaccinated patients. As this phase-I study demonstrated the safety and bioactivity of the treatment for RCC, a phase-II trial targeting minimal residual disease is currently under regulatory agency review in the USA [2]. Recently, another phase-I study of GM-CSF gene-transduced tumor vaccine for metastatic RCC patients was started by a multi-institutional group at the Institute of Medical Science, University of Tokyo, Japan.

Since immunotherapy has shown some clinical efficacy, current gene therapy approaches for RCC are mainly based on gene-modifed immunotherapy as listed in table 3 [22]. Several different strategies can be recognized in RCC protocols. Six protocols were based on a tumor vaccine strategy using in vitro gene-modified autologous cancer cells or partially HLA-matched allogeneic cancer cells. Four kinds of molecules, tumor necrosis factor, IL-2, GM-CSF and B7.1 (CD80) are being used to augment the host immunity. An additional protocol is planned to use IL-4-transduced autologous fibroblasts in combination with untransduced autologous tumors as a tumor vaccine. Other protocols use in vivo gene transfer strategies. The HLA-B7/β_2-microglobulin gene and IL-2 gene are being investigated in these protocols. Clinical trials using HLA-B7 are based on the results of preclinical studies which showed that the in vivo transduction of a gene encoding foreign MHC protein into an established tumor resulted in significant regression of parental tumor [23]. The generation of a CTL response against a parental tumor was demonstrated in this system [23]. At this time, although the side effects of gene-modified immunotherapy appear to be mild, the efficacy of this approach has yet to be proven. The optimal design and close immunological monitoring in these early trials may provide valuable information on future immunotherapy for RCC.

References

1 Roth JA, Cristiano RJ: Gene therapy for cancer: What have we done and where are we going? J Natl Cancer Inst 1997;88:21–39.

2 Simons JD, Marshall FF: The future of gene therapy in the treatment of urologic malignancies. Urol Clin North Am 1998;25:23–38.

3 Motzer RJ, Bander NH, Nanus DM: Renal-cell carcinoma. N Engl J Med 1996;335:865–875.

4 Figlin RA, Pierce WC, Kaboo R, Tso CL, Moldawer N, Gitlitz B, deKernion J, Belldegrun A: Treatment of metastatic renal cell carcinoma with nephrectomy, interleukin-2 and cytokine-primed or CD8(+) selected tumor infiltrating lymphocytes from primary tumor. J Urol 1997;158:740–745.

5 Pierce WC, Belldegrun A, Figlin RA: Cellular therapy: Scientific rationale and clinical results in the treatment of metastatic renal-cell carcinoma. Semin Oncol 1995;22:74–80.

6 Wang RF, Rosenberg SA: Human tumor antigens recognized by T lymphocytes: Implications for cancer therapy. J Leukoc Biol 1996;60:296–309.

7 Kawakami Y, Eliyahu S, Delgado CH, Robbins PF, Sakaguchi K, Appella E, Yannelli JR, Adema GJ, Miki T, Rosenberg SA: Identification of a human melanoma antigen recognized by tumor-infiltrating lymphocytes associated with in vivo tumor rejection. Proc Natl Acad Sci USA 1994;91: 6458–6462.

8 Rosenberg SA, Yang JC, White DE, Steinberg SM: Durabililty of complete responses in patients with metastatic cancer treated with high-dose interleukin-2: Identification of the antigens mediating response. Ann Surg 1998;228:307–319.

9 Gaugler B, Brouwenstijn N, Vantomme V, Szikora JP, Van der Spek CW, Patard JJ, Boon T, Schrier P, Van den Eynde BJ: A new gene coding for an antigen recognized by autologous cytolytic T lymphocytes on a human renal carcinoma. Immunogenetics 1996;44:323–330.

10 Brandle D, Brasseur F, Weynants P, Boon T, Van den Eynde BJ: A mutated HLA-A2 molecule recognized by autologous cytotoxic T lymphocytes on a human renal cell carcinoma. J Exp Med 1996;183:2501–2508.

11 Neumann E, Engelsberg A, Decker J, Storkel S, Jaeger E, Huber C, Seliger B: Heterogeneous expression of the tumor-associated antigens RAGE-1, PRAME, and Glycoprotein 75 in human renal cell carcinoma: Candidates for T-cell-based Immunotherapies? Cancer Res 1998;58:4090–4095.

12 Liu SQ, Kawai K, Shiraiwa H, Hayashi H, Akaza H, Hashizaki K, Shiba R, Saijo K, Ohono T: High rate of human autologous cytotoxic T lymphocytes against renal carcinoma cells culture with an interleukin cocktail. Jpn J Cancer Res 1998;89:1195–1201.

13 Chang AE, Aruga A, Cameran MJ, Sandak VK, Normolle DP, Fox BA, Shu S: Adoptive immunotherapy with vaccine-primed lymph node cells secondarily activated with anti-CD3 and interleukin-2. J Clin Oncol 1997;15:796–807.

14 Tepper RI, Mule JJ: Experimental and clinical studies of cytokine gene-modified tumor cells. Hum Gene Ther 1994;5:153–164.

15 Fearon ER, Pardoll DM, Itaya T, Golumbek P, Levitsky HI, Simons JW, Karasuyama H, Vogelstein B, Frost P: Interleukin-2 production by tumor cells bypasses T helper function in the generation of an antitumor response. Cell 1990;60:397–403.

16 Asher AL, Mule JJ, Kasid A, Restifo NP, Salo JC, Reichert CM, Jaffe G, Fendly B, Kriegler M, Rosenberg SA: Murine tumor cells transduced with the gene for tumor necrosis factor-α: Evidence for paracrine immune effects of tumor necrosis factor against tumors. J Immunol 1991;146:3227–3434.

17 Golumbek PT, Lazenby AJ, Levitsky HL, Jaffee LM, Karasuyama H, Baker M, Pardoll DM: Treatment of established renal cancer by tumor cells engineered to secrete interleukin-4. Science 1991;254:713–716.

18 Porgador A, Tzehoval E, Katz A, Vadai E, Revel M, Feldman M, Eisenbach L: Interleukin-6 gene transfection into Lewis lung carcinoma tumor cells suppresses the malignant phenotype and confers immunotherapeutic competence against parental metastatic cells. Cancer Res 1992;52:3679–3686.

19 Hock H, Dorsch M, Diamantstein T, Blankenstein T: Interleukin7 induces CD4+ T cell-dependent tumor rejection. J Exp Med 1991;174:1291–1298.

20 Dranoff G, Jaffee E, Lazenby A, Golumbek P, Levitsky H, Brose K, Jackson V, Hamada H, Pardoll D, Mulligan RC: Vaccination with irradiated tumor cells engineered to secrete murine granulocyte-macrophage colony-stimulating factor stimulates potent, specific, and long-lasting anti-tumor immunity. Proc Natl Acad Sci USA 1993;90:3539–3543.

21 Simons JW, Jaffee EM, Weber CE, Levitsky HI, Nelson WG, Carducci MA, Lazenby AW, Cohen LK, Finn CC, Clift SM, Hauda KM, Beck LA, Leiferman KM, Owens AH, Piantadosi S, Dranoff G, Mulligan RC, Pardoll DM, Marshall FF: Bioactivity of autologous irradiated renal cell carcinoma vaccine generated by ex vivo granulocyte-macrophage colony-stimulating factor gene transfer. Cancer Res 1997;57:1537–1546.

22 Human Gene Therapy Protocols: ORDA/NIH Internet Site: www.nih.gov/od/orda/protocol.htm.

23 Plautz GE, Yang Z, Wu B, Gao X, Huang L, Nabel GJ: Immunotherapy of malignancy by in vivo gene transfer into tumors. Proc Natl Acad Sci USA 1990;90:4645–4649.

Koji Kawai, MD, Department of Urology, Institute of Clinical Medicine, University of Tsukuba, 1-1-1 Tennodai, Tsukuba City, Ibaraki 305 (Japan)
Tel./Fax +81 298 53 3223

Hino O (ed): Kidney Cancer. Recent Results of Basic and Clinical Research.
Contrib Nephrol. Basel, Karger, 1999, vol 128, pp 82–98

Wilms' Tumor (Nephroblastoma)

Kinji Yokomori

Department of Pediatric Surgery, Japanese Red Cross Medical Center, Tokyo, Japan

Epidemiology

Tumors of the kidney in children comprise both malignant ones, such as Wilms' tumor (or nephroblastoma, 90%), clear cell sarcoma (3%) and rhabdoid tumor (2%), and a rather benign one, mesoblastic nephroma (2%). Very rarely were cases of adult-type malignancy, adenocarcinoma (renal cell carcinoma, <1%), reported.

The frequency of Wilms' tumor varies from race to race; the incidence is three times higher in Blacks than East Asians, and that in Whites is intermediate, between the two extremes [1]. It occurs with approximately equal frequency in both sexes except for the tumor associated with anaplasia (see below; twice as common in females), and with an incidence peak between 1 and 3 years of age.

Associated Congenital Anomalies and Syndromatic Conditions

An important feature of Wilms' tumor is its association with congenital anomalies in approximately 15% of children with this tumor, the most common being genitourinary anomalies (4.4%), hemihypertrophy (2.9%), and sporadic aniridia (1.1%) [2]. The common defects in the genitourinary tract are horseshoe kidney, hypospadias, cryptorchidism, renal dysplasia, and duplicated collecting system. Hemihypertrophy is the most prominent among the musculoskeletal anomalies including clubfoot, rib fusion, phocomelia and hip dislocation.

Wilms' tumor has been shown in association with several uncommon, albeit distinct syndromes, as well as conditions with increased risk of this

Table 1. Syndromatic conditions associated with increased risk of Wilms' tumor

WAGR syndrome
Beckwith-Wiedemann syndrome
Denys-Drash syndrome
Perlman syndrome
Klippel-Trenaunay syndrome
Simpson-Golabi-Behmel syndrome
Bloom syndrome
Poland syndrome
Down syndrome
Marfan syndrome
Sotos syndrome
Dandy-Walker syndrome
De Lange syndrome
Fanconi syndrome
Neurofibromatosis
Ataxia-telangiectasia
Tuberous sclerosis
Chromosomal anomalies (trisomy 8, 13)

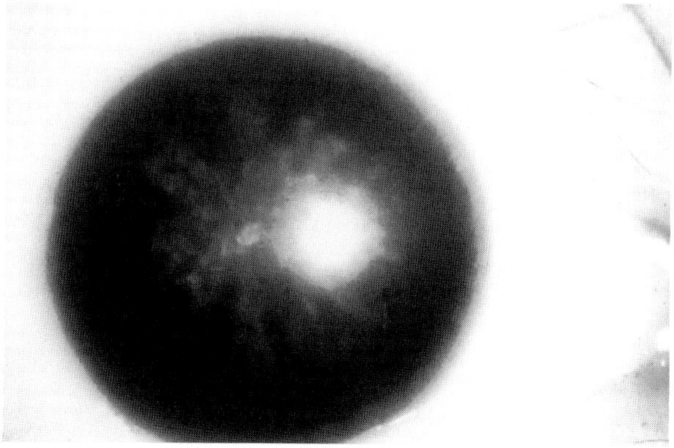

Fig. 1. Aniridia in a 3-year-old boy with WGAR syndrome.

tumor (table 1). The patients with the WAGR syndrome (Wilms' tumor, aniridia (fig. 1), genitourinary anomalies, and mental retardation) have a consistent deletion in chromosome 11p13 of their somatic cells [3]. The Beckwith-Wiedemann syndrome (BWS; fig. 2) is made up of umbilical anomalies (omphalocele or umbilical hernia), macroglossia, and macrosomia (neonatal gigantism, post-

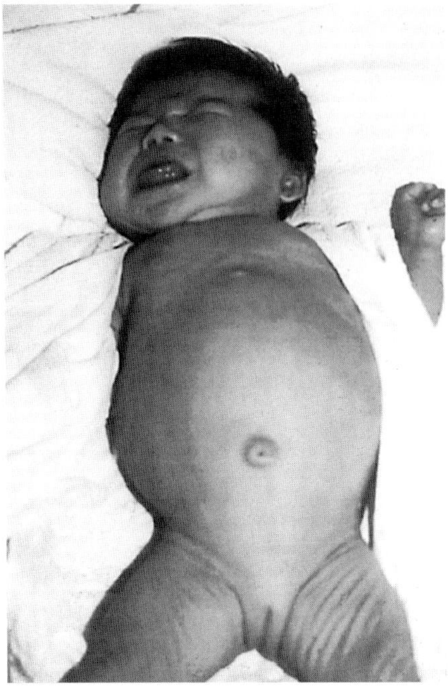

Fig. 2. Appearance of a newborn baby with Beckwith-Wiedemann syndrome.

natal overgrowth, or hemihypertrophy) [4, 5], and the patients with this syndrome are known to be at higher risk for Wilms' tumor, hepatoblastoma, and adrenocortical tumor [6]. Constitutional karyotype analysis has mapped the BWS locus to chromosome 11p15 [7]. Children with pseudohermaphroditism (fig. 3) and renal glomerulopathies (glomerulonephritis or nephrotic syndrome) may develop Wilms' tumor, constituting the Denys-Drash syndrome, which is associated with point mutations within chromosome 11p13, similar to those in the WAGR syndrome [8].

Etiology

In 1972 Knudson and Strong [9] proposed a genetic model for the development of Wilms' tumor based on the two-event hypothesis, predicting that all Wilms' tumors develop as a consequence of two mutational events in a tumor-suppressor gene(s). They believed that children at risk for Wilms' tumor were born with a constitutional DNA mutation (the first event) in one allele of a presumed tumor-suppressor gene. The second event in the other allele results in tumorigenesis, and the tumor is potentially hereditary and could be multicentric in origin. By contrast, the sporadic form results from two somatic

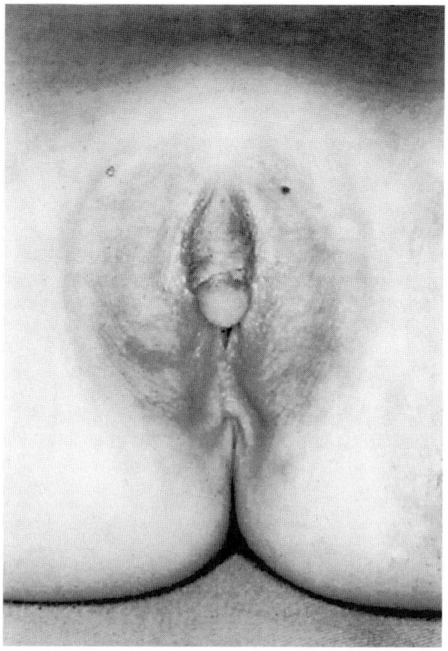

Fig. 3. Genital appearance of a 2-year-old boy with Denys-Drash syndrome.

mutations in a single cell, and affected children are unlikely to develop multiple tumors, since the two events are unlikely to occur independently in more than one cell. Subsequently this two-event inactivation of a tumor-suppressor gene for at least two different genetic loci has been confirmed. In many cases, the first event inactivates one allele by way of mutation in the gene itself, whereas the second hit inactivates the other allele by way of deletion, which is detected by loss of heterozygosity. However, the genetic events responsible for the development of Wilms' tumor seem more complex than those leading to the occurrence of retinoblastoma.

The constitutional deletion in the short arm of one copy of chromosome 11 at band 13 in children with the WAGR syndrome, demonstrated by karyotypic analysis [10], provided the first clue to the location of a gene responsible for Wilms' tumor formation, and led to the independent identification of the first Wilms' tumor-suppressor gene, called *WT1*, at 11p13 by three groups in 1990 [11–13]. The WAGR deletion was further shown to encompass a number of contiguous genes other than *WT1*, including the aniridia gene called *PAX6*. The *WT1* consists of ten axons encoding for a protein with a molecular weight of 45–49 kD, depending on the presence or absence of two alternative splicing events. Based on the presence of four zinc-finger domains, a motif specific to DNA binding, at the carboxyl terminus, and of a domain rich in proline and glutamine, a motif characteristic of transcriptional factors, at the amino

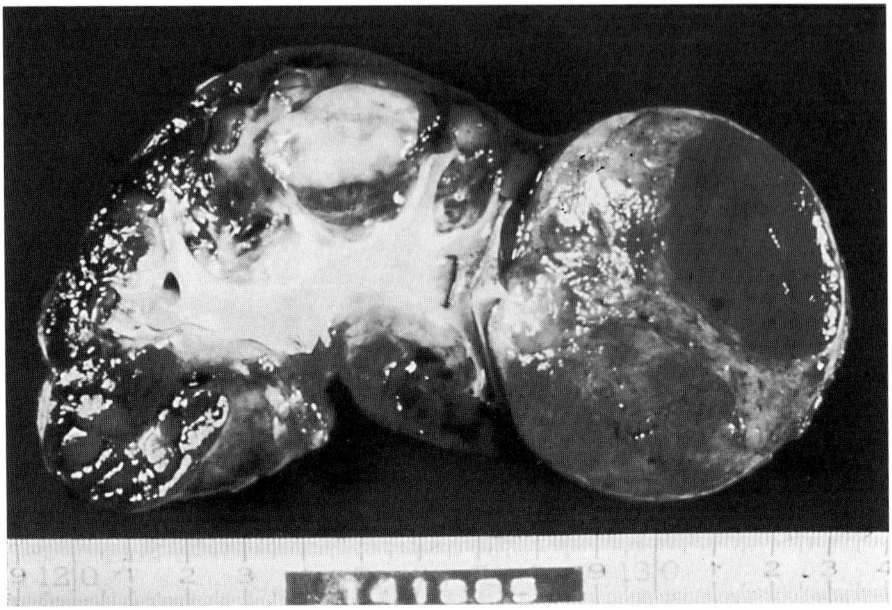

Fig. 4. Gross appearance of the cut surface of a Wilms' tumor.

terminus, the WT1 protein is viewed to regulate the transcription of other genes. Candidate genes for the target of the WT1 protein include insulin-like growth factor II [14], and the early growth response gene, *PAX2* [15]. The WT1 protein plays an important role in genitourinary tract organogenesis, as expected from a variety of severe genitourinary anomalies seen in the WAGR syndrome and the Denys-Drash syndrome. Approximately 30–40% of Wilms tumors manifest loss of heterozygosity for the *WT1* locus, and only 10% of the patients were reported to have *WT1* mutations identified [16].

Children with BWS develop embryonal tumors with increased frequency, with the Wilms' tumor being the most frequent. As reported by Sotelo-Avila [6] 17 of 200 BWS patients developed malignant tumors, among which 10 were Wilms' tumors. Genetic linkage analyses and studies on uniparental paternal isodisomy for 11p15 suggested that the locus for BWS maps to chromosome 11p15 [17, 18]. Further study on a subset of Wilms' tumor demonstrated tumor-specific loss of heterozygosity for markers telomeric of 11p13 with maintenance of heterozygosity for 11p13 loci [19], suggesting a second independent Wilms' tumor-suppressor gene, the putative *WT2*, at 11p15. The *WT2* locus at 11p15 may well explain the above-mentioned association of Wilms' tumor with the BWS, but at this moment it remains unknown whether the BWS gene and *WT2* are identical or not. In tumors with loss of

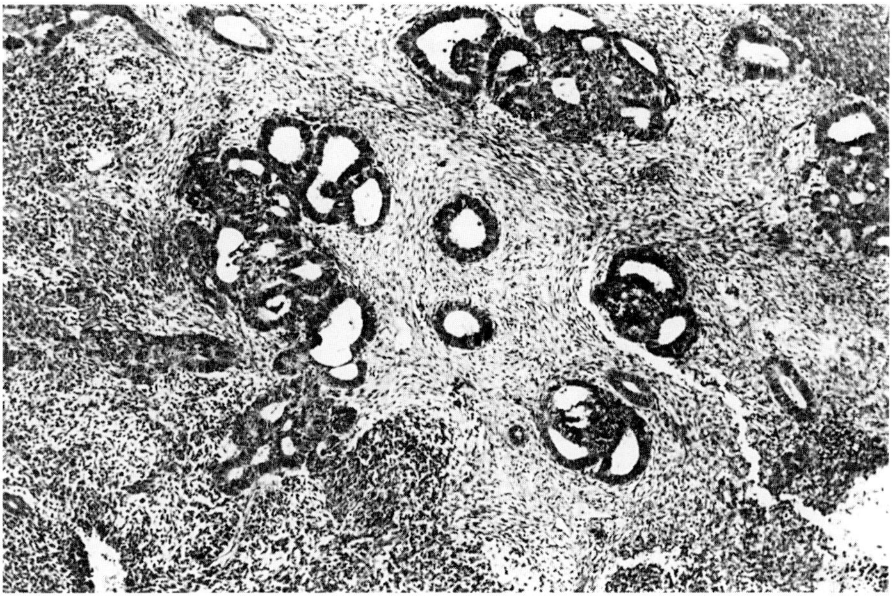

Fig. 5. Typical microscopic appearance of a Wilms' tumor showing a triphasic pattern.

heterozygosity, the maternal allele at 11p15 was invariably lost [20], suggesting the 11p15 loci are subject to genomic imprinting. Two candidate genes for *WT2*, insulin-like growth factor II (*IGF2*) gene and another tumor-suppressor gene at a locus adjacent to *IGF2, H19*, are recognized. IGF2 is an embryonal growth factor, which is highly expressed in Wilms' tumor tissues. The *IGF2* gene is imprinted, with only the paternal allele being expressed [21]. The *H19* gene is also imprinted, but only the maternal allele is active [22].

In familial Wilms' tumor cases, which account for only 2% of all, neither WT1 nor WT2 was implicated [23], suggesting the presence of a third as yet unidentified Wilms' tumor gene.

Pathology

Gross Appearance

Wilms' tumor is usually a spherical growth that occurs in any part of the kidney on either side, and deforms or effaces the renal contour. The tumor is sharply demarcated from the adjacent renal parenchyma by a 'pseudocapsule'. On bisection, the tumor tends to bulge from the cut surface, and has a uniform, pale gray or tan appearance and a soft consistency (fig. 4). Prominent septae

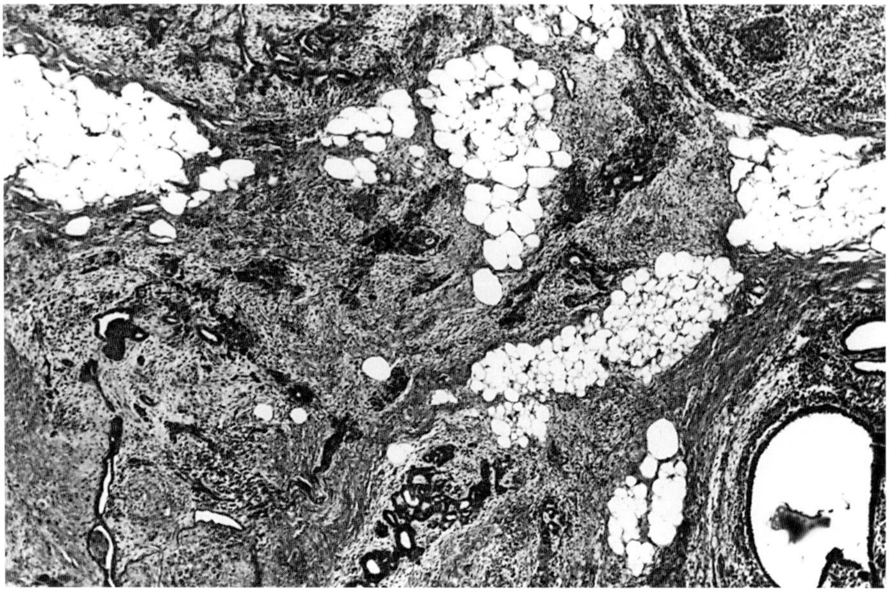

Fig. 6. Mesenchymal derivatives seen in the tumor from a WAGR patient.

subdividing the tumor tissue into lobules, polypoid protrusions of tumor into the pelvicaliceal system, areas of hemorrhage and cystic spaces of various sizes may be seen. Hyperplastic nephrogenic rests, the percursor lesions of Wilms' tumor which are visible by the naked eye, are sometimes seen at the periphery of the tumor and/or beneath the renal capsule covering the residual renal parenchyma uninvolved by the tumor (see below). Among the cases registered by the National Wilms' Tumor Study (NWTS) in the USA, 7.0% were multicentric and 5.4% were bilateral in origin [24].

Microscopic Appearance

Three Basic Components

The classic Wilms' tumor is composed of three basic components, i.e. undifferentiated cells (blastema), epithelial structures (tubules and glomeruloid bodies), and the intervening stroma, showing a triphasic pattern (fig. 5). The stroma may include mesenchymal derivatives such as striated muscle, adipose tissue, osteoid and cartilage (fig. 6). These components can occur in any proportion, exhibiting a highly variable histologic appearance. In some rare occasions, on the contrary, one-sided differentiation may give rise to a mono-

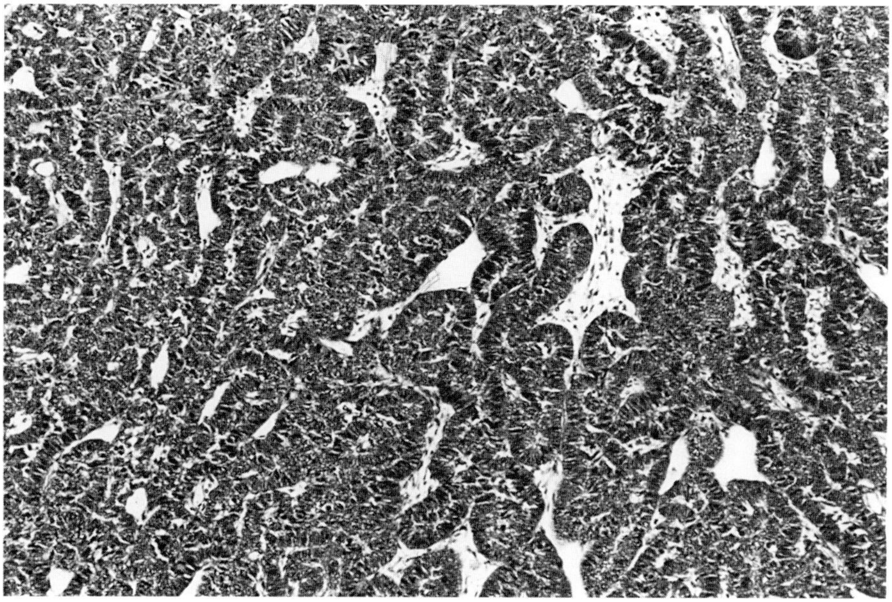

Fig. 7. Monophasic epithelial Wilms' tumor.

phasic Wilms' tumor, which may consist solely of blastemal or epithelial (fig. 7) or mesenchymal components.

Anaplastic Wilms' Tumor

Wilms' tumor with foci of anaplasia is classified as a tumor of unfavorable histology (UH), and the patient's prognosis is significantly poorer than that of the patient with a tumor of favorable histology (FH), i.e. without anaplasia. Anaplasia is defined by the NWTS Pathology Center as the presence of cells with threefold nuclear enlargement, hyperchromatism, and bizarre mitotic figures [25] (fig. 8). These anaplastic changes may be confined to sharply demarcated foci ('focal anaplasia'), or widely scattered through the tumor ('diffuse anaplasia'), with the latter having a worse prognosis [26].

Anaplasia is found in about 5% of cases, and with a higher incidence in female patients. It is rarely seen in tumors of patients younger than 2 years of age at diagnosis, but its presence increases with the age of the patient. Anaplastic Wilms' tumors frequently show aneuploidy [27] and have frequent mutations in the tumor-suppressor gene p53 [28].

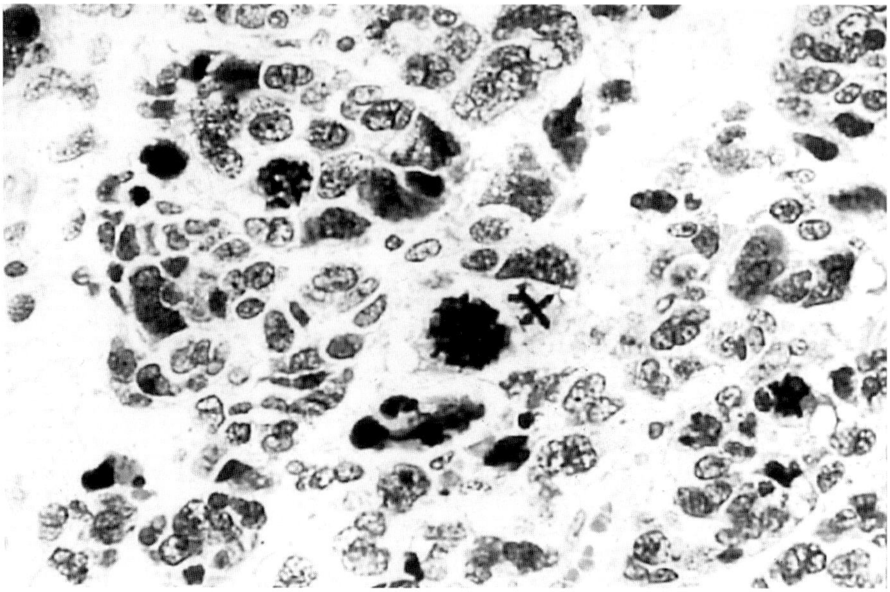

Fig. 8. Cells exhibiting features of anaplasia.

Nephrogenic Rests

Nephrogenic rests (NRs) are foci of immature blastemic cells, which are found in approximately 1% of routine postmortem examinations in infants [29]. These lesions have also been encountered in 25–40% of children with sporadic Wilms' tumor [30]; the rests are often found within the residual kidney at the periphery of the nearby expanding tumor. A report that, in 2 children with Wilms' tumor associated with NRs, the same somatic mutation of *WT1* was detected both in the tumor and the rests [31] molecular biologically supported the long-harbored speculation that NRs may be premalignant lesions of Wilms' tumor.

Two distinctive subtypes of NRs are known, depending on their anatomical location within the renal parenchyma (fig. 9). The rests found at the periphery of the renal lobe are called perilobar NRs (fig. 10), and those located deep in the renal medulla are called intralobar NRs (fig. 11). Tumors in association with perilobar NRs are usually composed of three basic components, i.e. nodules or cords of blastema, tubules and glomeruloid bodies, and the surrounding stroma, without any mesenchymal derivatives, and frequently occur in BWS patients, whereas intralobar NR-associated tumors are abundant in mesenchymal derivatives, and develop in children with WAGR syndrome and Denys-Drash syndrome.

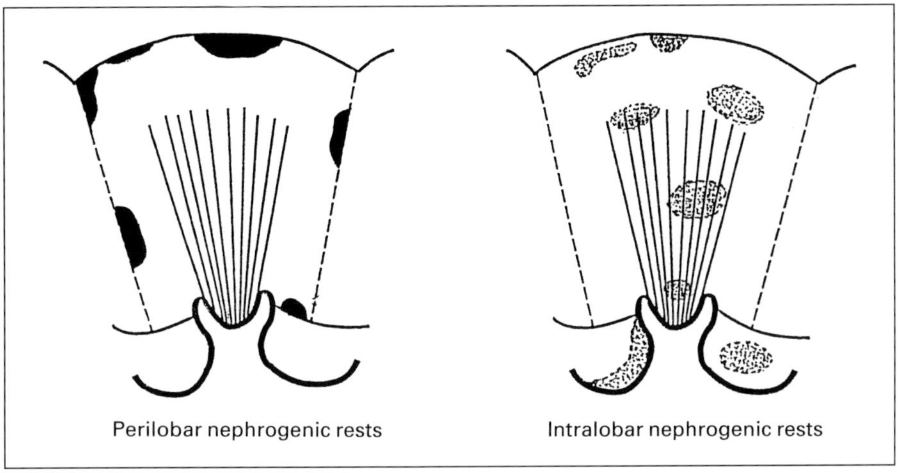

Fig. 9. Schematic illustration showing anatomical locations of perilobar and intralobar nephrogenic rests within the renal lobe.

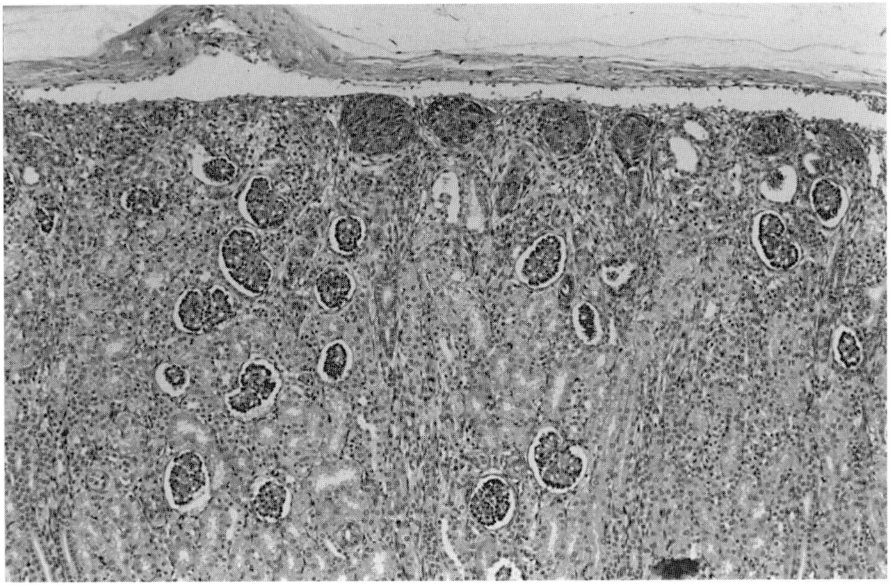

Fig. 10. Perilobar nephrogenic rests beneath the renal capsule.

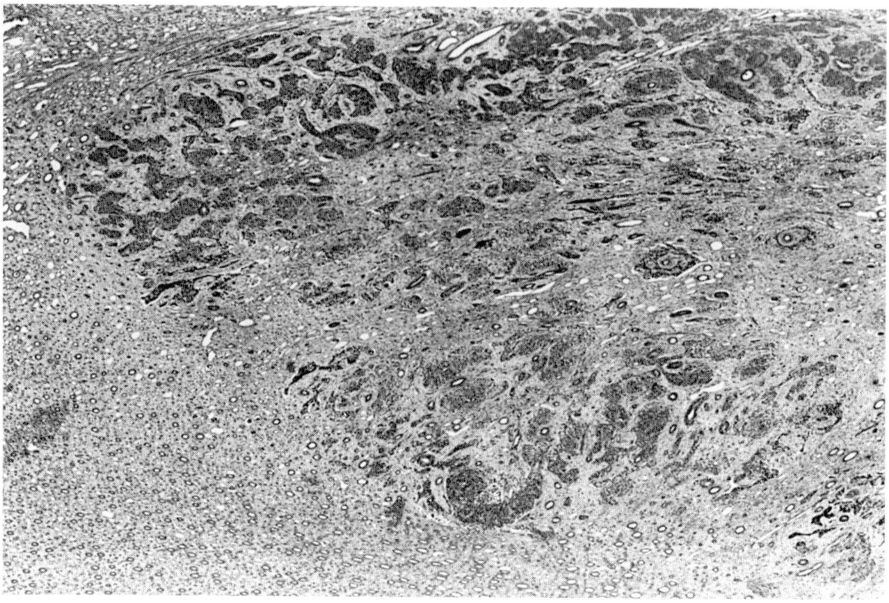

Fig. 11. Intralobar nephrogenic rests compressed by the expanding tumor at the tumor-kidney junction.

Clinical Manifestations

Wilms' tumor is often recognized by a family member as an asymptomatic abdominal mass (fig. 12), although abdominal pain, hematuria, fever, malaise, weight loss, anemia are common. Hypertension is present in 1 of 4 patients, due mainly to ectopic renin production by the tumor tissue [32], and partly to the renal artery ischemia caused by the tumor compression. It is also important to pay attention to signs of congenital anomalous syndromes associated with Wilms' tumor, as listed in table 1.

Laboratory Findings

At this moment no diagnostic blood or urine tests for the definitive diagnosis of Wilms' tumor are available. Lactate dehydrogenase levels in serum are usually elevated with abnormal isozyme patterns, but these are not specific to Wilms' tumor. Serum levels of inactive renin (prorenin) may be made use of as a tumor marker for Wilms' tumor [33]. Determination of basic fibroblast growth factor in the urine may reflect the course of the tumor [34]. The tumor

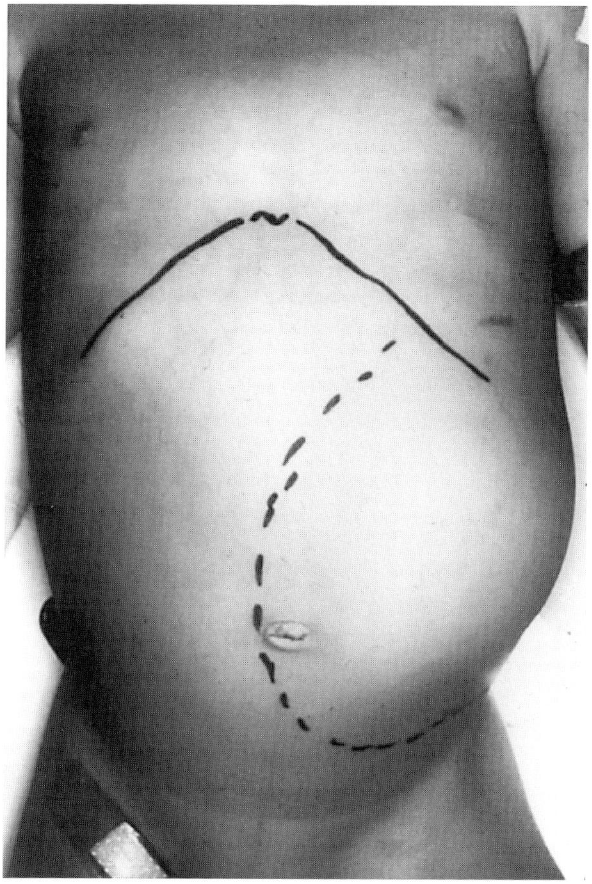

Fig. 12. Bulging abdomen of a 2-year-old girl with a Wilms' tumor in the right kidney.

may produce erythropoietin, leading to polycythemia, secondary hypercalcemia, and a clinical picture similar to von Willebrand disease.

Diagnostic Imaging Studies

Plain X-ray films of the abdomen may reveal a mass contour in the flank and displacement of bowel shadows to the opposite side. Plain chest radiographs may detect pulmonary metastases. Excretory urography (intravenous pyelography, IVP) has long been employed worldwide, revealing distortion and displacement of the pelvicalyceal and collecting systems (fig. 13).

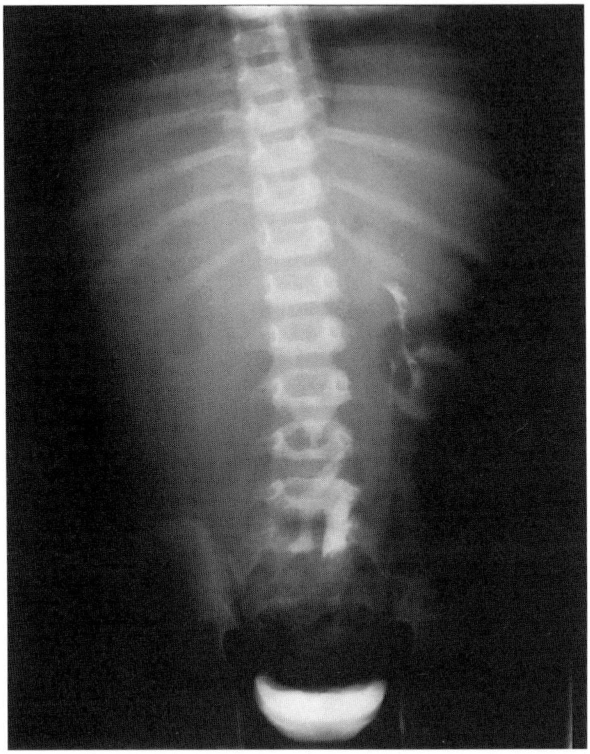

Fig. 13. Intravenous pyelogram shows distortion of the right-sided pelvicalyceal system.

Now IVP has gradually been replaced by the less invasive imaging modalities, such as CT scan, MRI and ultrasonography. CT of the abdomen may visualize the tumor(s) and/or NRs in the affected kidney, as well as those lesions in the contralateral kidney (fig. 14). MRI also shows the pattern of heterogenous tissues within the tumor. Real-time ultrasonography can detect tumor thrombi in the renal vein, the inferior vena cava and the right atrium. Other imaging studies include a radionuclide bone scan and X-ray skeletal survey for the bone lesions.

Staging

With regard to tumor spread, each tumor is clinically staged according to the staging criteria. The staging system most frequently used is that of the NWTS group (table 2). The extent of local disease is determined at the time of surgery, and confirmed by the pathologist who determines the presence or absence of anaplasia within the tumor.

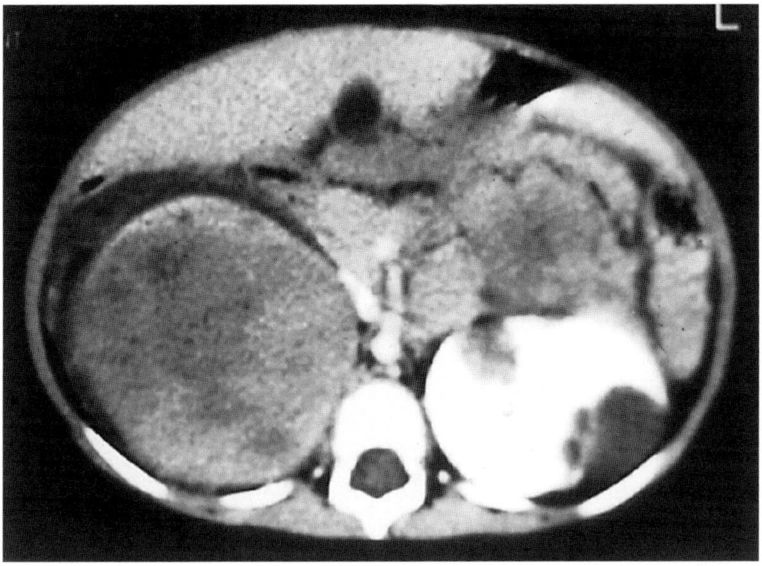

Fig. 14. Abdominal CT shows a huge Wilms' tumor in the right kidney and the hyperplastic intralobar nephrogenic rests in the left kidney.

Table 2. Staging system of Wilms tumor (NWTS)

Stage I	Tumor limited to kidney, completely excised Capsular surface intact; no tumor rupture; no residual tumor Apparent beyond margins of excision
Stage II	Tumor extends beyond kidney but is completely excised Regional extension of tumor; vessel infiltration; tumor biopsied or local spillage of tumor confined to the flank No residual tumor apparent at or beyond margins of excision.
Stage III	Residual non-hematogenous tumor confined to the abdomen Lymph node involvement of hilus, perisortic chains or beyond; diffuse peritoneal contamination by tumor spillage; peritoneal implants of tumor; tumor extends beyond surgical margins either microscopically or macroscopically; tumor not completely removable because of local infiltration into vital structures
Stage IV	Deposits beyond stage III (e.g. lung, liver, bone, brain)
Stage V	Bilateral renal involvement at diagnosis

Treatment

Therapy for Wilms' tumor is one of the great success stories in modern oncology. Currently two different therapeutic approaches, preoperative and postoperative treatments, are being employed. Postoperative treatment is the method most often advocated worldwide including the NWTS group [35], whereas preoperative treatment has been used by the International Society of Pediatric Oncology group in Europe in a series of clinical trials [36]. In both approaches, similar combined chemotherapeutic regimens have been adopted, with only the timing and indications for surgery, radio- and chemotherapy differing from each other. Dactinomycin and vincristine are the most effective drugs for most of cases with a FH, and are used in conjunction with surgery, without radiotherapy, for all stage-I and II tumors with FH. Stage-I tumors with an UH are similarly treated, but UH tumors with stages II–V are treated by more toxic chemotherapeutic agents and radiotherapy. Doxorubicin is a significant addition to the treatment of patients with advanced disease. Pulmonary irradiation and three-drug combination chemotherapy are now recommended for most patients with stage-IV disease. Preoperative therapy is generally indicated for patients with bilateral tumors (stage V) to facilitate eventual renal salvage procedures. This approach preserves renal parenchyma and optimizes renal function without compromising survival.

Prognosis

The most significant prognostic variables are histologic subtype (FH vs. UH) and stage. As the majority of Wilms' tumors are at low stages and of FH, the overall 2-year survival is better than 85% with either pre- or postoperative treatment [35, 36]. A favorable outcome was observed even among tumors with focal anaplasia, with the 2-year survival being as good as 85%, but it was no more than 50% for diffuse anaplasia [37].

References

1 Stiller CA, Parkin DM: International variations in the incidence of childhood renal tumors. Br J Cancer 1990;62:1026–1030.

2 Pendergrass TW: Congenital anomalies in children with Wilms' tumor: A new survey. Cancer 1976; 37:404–408.

3 Miller RW, Fraumeni JF, Manning MD: Association of Wilms' tumor with aniridia, hemihypertrophy and other congenital anomalies. N Engl J Med 1964;270:922–927.

4 Beckwith JB: Extreme cytomegaly of the adrenal fetal cortex, omphalocele, hyperplasia of the kidneys and pancreas, and Leidig-cell hyperplasia: Another syndrome? Presented to the Western Society for Pediatric Research, Los Angeles, 1963.

5 Wiedemann HR: Complexe malformatif familial avec hernie ombilicale et macroglossie – un syndrome nouveau? J Génét Hum 1964;13:223–232.
6 Sotelo-Avila CI: Complete and incomplete form of Beckwith-Wiedemann syndrome: Their oncologic potential. J Pediatr 1980;76:585–589.
7 Turleau C, DeGrouchy J: Beckwith-Wiedemann syndrome clinical comparison between patients with and without 11p15 trisomy. Ann Genet 1985;28:93–96.
8 Coppes MJ, Huff V, Pelletier J: Denys-Drash syndrome: Relating a clinical disorder to genetic alterations in the tumor suppressor gene WT1. J Pediatr 1993;123:673.
9 Knudson AG, Strong LC: Mutation and cancer: A model for Wilms' tumor of the kidney. J Natl Cancer Inst 1972;48:313–324.
10 Riccardi VM, Sujansky E, Smith AC, Francke U: Chromosomal imbalance in the aniridia-Wilms' tumor association: 11p interstitial deletion. Pediatrics 1978;61:604–610.
11 Call KM, Glaser T, Ito CY, Buckler AJ, Pelletier J, Haber DA, Rose EA, Kral A, Yeger H, Lewis WH, Jones C, Housman DE: Isolation and characterization of a zinc finger polypeptide gene at the human chromosome 11 Wilms' tumor locus. Cell 1990;60:509–520.
12 Gessler M, Poustka A, Cavenee W, Neve RL, Orkin SH, Bruns GAP: Homozygous deletion on Wilms tumors of a zinc-finger gene identified by chromosome jumping. Nature 1990;343:774–778.
13 Bonetta L, Kuehn SE, Huang A, Law DJ, Kalikin LM, Koi M, Reeve AE, Brownstein BH, Yeger H, William BRG, Feinberg AP: Wilms' tumor locus on 11p13 defined by multiple CpG island-associated transcripts. Science 1990;250:994–997.
14 Drummond IA: Repression of the insulin-like growth factor II gene by the Wilms' tumor suppressor WT1. Science 1992;256:674–678.
15 Tagge EP: Paired box gene expression in Wilms' tumor. J Pediatr Surg 1994;29:134–141.
16 Huff V, Miwa H, Haber DA, Housman D, Strong LC, Saunders GF: Evidence for WT1 as a Wilms' tumor (WT) gene: Intragenic germinal deletion in bilateral WT. Am J Hum Genet 1991;48:997–1003.
17 Koufos A, Grundy P, Morgan K, Aleck KA, Hadro T, Lampkin BC, Kalbakji A, Cavenee WK: Familial Wiedemann-Beckwith syndrome and a second Wilms' tumor locus both map to 11p15.5. Am J Hum Genet 1989;44:711–719.
18 Henry I, Bonaiti-Pellie C, Chehensse V, Beldjord C, Schwartz C, Utermann G, Junien C: Uniparental paternal disomy in a genetic cancer-predisposing syndrome. Nature 1991;351:665–667.
19 Coppes MJ, Haber DA, Grundy PE: Genetic events in the development of Wilms' tumor. N Engl J Med 1994;331:586–590.
20 Schroeder WT, Chao L-Y, Dao DD, Strong LC, Pathak S, Riccardi V, Lewis WH, Saunders GF: Nonrandom loss of maternal chromosome 11 alleles in Wilms' tumors. 1987;40:413–420.
21 Rainier S, Johnson LA, Dobry CJ, Ping AJ, Grundy PE, Feinberg AP: Relaxation of imprinted genes in human cancer. Nature 1993;362:747–749.
22 Steenman MJ, Rainier S, Dobry CJ, Grundy P, Horon IL, Feinberg AP: Loss of imprinting of IGF2 is linked to reduced expression and abnormal methylation of H19 in Wilms tumor. Nat Genet 1994;7:433–439.
23 Grundy P, Koufos A, Morgan M, Li FP, Meadows AT, Cavenee WK: Familial predisposition to Wilms tumor does not map to the short arm of chromosome 11. Nature 1988;336:374–376.
24 Breslow N, Beckwith JB, Ciol M, Sharples K: Age distribution of Wilms' tumor: Report from the National Wilms Tumor Study. Cancer Res 1988;48:1653–1657.
25 Bonadio JF, Storer B, Norkool P, Farewell VT, Beckwith JB, D'Angio GJ: Anaplastic Wilms' tumor: Clinical and pathological studies. J Clin Oncol 1985;3:513–520.
26 Faria P, Beckwith JB: A new definition of focal anaplasia identifies cases with good outcome. A report from the National Wilms' Tumor Study (abstract). Mod Pathol 1993;6:3.
27 Re GG: Nephroblastoma (Wilms' tumor): A model system of aberrant renal development. Semin Diagn Pathol 1994;11:126–135.
28 Bardeesy N: Anaplastic Wilms' tumor, a subtype displaying poor prognosis, harbours p53 gene mutations. Nat Genet 1994;7:91–97.
29 Bennington JL, Beckwith JB: Tumor of the kidney, renal pelvis, and ureter; in Atlas of Tumor Pathology, Ser 2, Fasc 12. Washington, Armed Forces Institute of Pathology, 1975, pp 31–78.

30 Beckwith JB, Kiviat NB, Bonadio JF: Nephrogenic rests, nephroblastomatosis, and the pathogenesis of Wilms' tumor. Pediatr Pathol 1990;10:1–36.
31 Park S, Bernard A, Bove KE, Sens DA, Hazen-Martin DJ, Garvin AJ, Haber DA: Inactivation of WT1 in nephrogenic rests, genetic precursors to Wilms' tumor. Nat Genet 1993;5:363–367.
32 Yokomori K, Hori T, Takemura T, Tsuchida Y: Demonstration of both primary and secondary reninism in renal tumors in children. J Pediatr Surg 1988;23:403–409.
33 Johnson MA, Carachi R, Lindop GB, Leckie B: Inactive renin levels in recurrent nephroblastoma. J Pediatr Surg 1991;26:613–614.
34 Argenta PA, Lin RY, Sullivan KM: Basic fibroblast growth factor is a Wilms' tumor marker. Surg Forum 1994;45:789.
35 Green DM, Breslow NE, Evans I, Moksness J, Finklestein JZ, Evans AE, D'Angio GJ: The effect of chemotherapy dose intensity on the hematological toxicity of the treatment for Wilms' tumor. A report from the National Wilms' Tumor Study. Am J Pediatr Hematol Oncol 1994;16:207–212.
36 Delemarre JF, Sandstedt B, Gerard-Marchant G: SIOP nephroblastoma trials and studies, morphological aspects; in Raybaud C (ed): Pediatric Oncology. Amsterdam, Excerpta Medica, 1982, pp 261–272.
37 D'Angio GJ, Breslow N, Beckwith JB, Evans A, Baum H, deLorimier A, Fernbach D, Hrabovsky E, Jones B, Kelalis P: Treatment of Wilms' tumor. Results of the 3rd National Wilms' Tumor Study. Cancer 1989;64:347–360.

Kinji Yokomori, MD, Department of Pediatric Surgery, Japanese Red Cross Medical Center, Tokyo (Japan)

Hino O (ed): Kidney Cancer. Recent Results of Basic and Clinical Research.
Contrib Nephrol. Basel, Karger, 1999, vol 128, pp 99–125

Pathogenesis of Renal Cell Adenomas and Carcinomas in Animal Models

P. Bannasch, H. Zerban

Division of Cell Pathology, Deutsches Krebsforschungszentrum, Heidelberg, Germany

Introduction

Renal neoplasms rarely develop spontaneously in laboratory animals, but have been induced in different species, particularly in small rodents, by a variety of oncogenic agents including chemicals, hormones, radiation and viruses [1–5]. Although more than 100 chemicals, different types of high-energy radiation and viruses have been identified as renal carcinogens in rodents, only a few animal models of renal carcinogenesis have been analyzed in greater detail. The main reason for this selective approach seems to be that phenotypic similarities rather than differences are characteristic of neoplastic development induced by the various oncogenic agents [1]. A hereditary renal cell carcinoma was described in rats by Eker [6] and has been thoroughly studied as a model of dominantly inherited predisposition to a specific tumor type [7–9]. Even if such genetic events are involved in the evolution of renal cell carcinomas, phenotypic similarities with certain types of tumors induced by exogenous agents are obvious [9, 10].

The spectrum of renal neoplasms observed in animal models is nearly as broad as that known from human pathology [4]. Whereas experience in human pathology has guided the classification and histogenetic derivation of experimental renal tumors for a long time, several experimental findings had a strong impact on the classification and elucidation of the pathogenesis of human kidney tumors in the past two decades [1, 4, 5].

As to the variety of etiologic agents producing renal neoplasms the reader is referred to a number of reviews [1–5, 11, 12]. This article will be focused on some animal models which have significantly contributed to our understanding of the pathogenesis of renal neoplasms, especially renal cell adenomas and carcinomas which predominate in both experimental and human renal carcinogenesis. In most of these animal models, neoplastic development in the kidney takes a long time; in the rat, this lag period often lasts for 1 or 2 years.

Classification

Experimental renal cell tumors are usually classified as adenomas including oncocytomas, and carcinomas [1, 13–15]. The main site of origin of renal cell tumors is the renal cortex, but they may also develop from the outer medulla, and should, therefore, not be designated as cortical epithelial tumors [5]. As in human pathology, in many cases in rodents an unequivocal distinction between adenomas and carcinomas is difficult, if not impossible, on morphological grounds. Whereas small lesions are frequently grouped with adenomas, large tumors are classified as carcinomas, particularly when cellular atypia, necrosis or invasion of the adjacent tissue is evident [14]. A high propensity for distant metastases, especially to the lungs, has been reported for renal cell tumors exceeding 2 cm in diameter [16, 17]. An exceptional case is the oncocytoma which, at least in the rat, always appears to behave as a benign neoplasm [13].

Using cytomorphological and simple cytochemical criteria we have introduced a new classification of renal cell tumors which had been induced in rats by N-nitrosomorpholine, more than two decades ago [18–21]. In addition to oncocytomas, basophilic, chromophobic, acidophilic, and clear/acidophilic (granular) cell tumors were distinguished. This classification has not only proved suitable for both spontaneous and induced renal cell tumors in rodents [1, 5], but also prompted Thoenes et al. [22, 23] to propose a new classification of human renal cell tumors, separating chromophobic, chromophilic (including granular), and clear cell carcinomas from oncocytomas, which has been widely accepted in the meantime [24, 25]. A detailed listing of the experimental production of the different types of rat renal cell tumors has been provided elsewhere [14], but N-nitrosomorpholine which has been shown to induce all types of rat renal cell tumors [14, 26] may not be an exception since a similar situation has recently been reported for N-ethyl-N-hydroxyethylnitrosamine [27].

All rodent renal cell tumors develop from the renal tubular system. The main determinant for the type of tumor induced appears to be the specific differentiation of the target cell rather than the oncogenic agent [1, 5, 26, 27]. It is, hence, important to realize that the renal tubular system is a complex structure comprising a number of physiologically well-defined segments, each

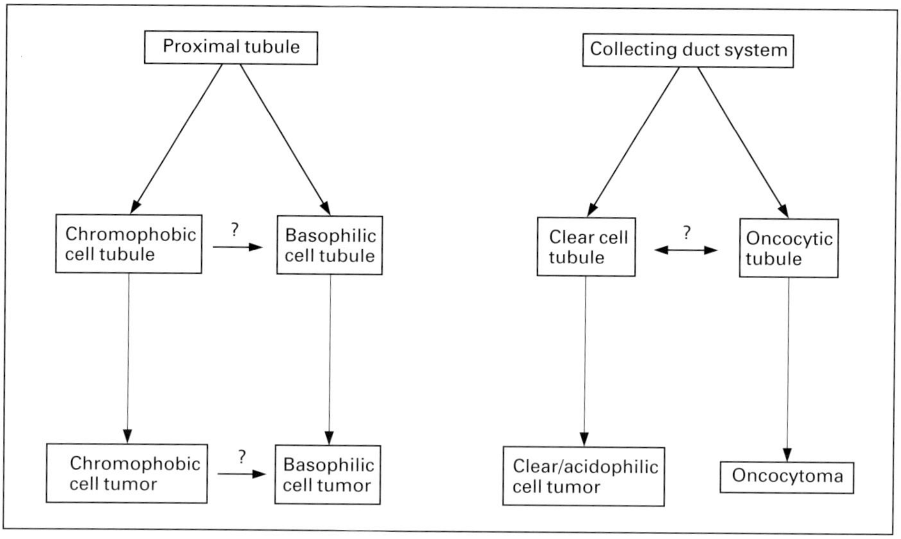

Fig. 1. Sites of origin and developmental stages of different types of renal cell tumor. From Bannasch and Zerban [1].

of which is lined by specifically differentiated cells [28]. The various types of renal cell tumor apparently develop from different segments of this system (fig. 1), particularly from the proximal tubule and the collecting duct system [5, 27, 29]. Specific cellular changes within these tubular segments regularly precede the manifestation of the renal cell tumors by weeks and months.

A confusing variety of terms has been proposed for such preneoplastic tubular lesions [12], including 'atypical tubule' [30], 'dysplastic tubule' [31, 32], 'simple tubular hyperplasia' [33, 34], and 'atypical tubular hyperplasia' [30, 34], the latter being considered as a more advanced stage of neoplastic development. All these collective nouns confuse rather than clarify the situation. Thus, it is evident that an 'atypical tubule' composed of basophilic cells differs from a tubule lined by clear cells, and particularly by oncocytes, in its potential to progress to a neoplasm [1, 26]. All types of preneoplastic tubules consist of cells markedly altered in their morphology and intermediate metabolism, whereas the term 'hyperplasia' indicates a proliferation of normal cells under conditions of reparative or compensatory regeneration [14]. We, therefore, prefer to maintain the designation of the preneoplastic tubules using the altered cell types as descriptors, e.g. clear cell tubule, basophilic cell tubule, and oncocytic tubule [19–21]. This descriptive terminology appears to be most appropriate because it does not anticipate the biological behavior of the respective lesions, but permits the development of an ever-increasing number

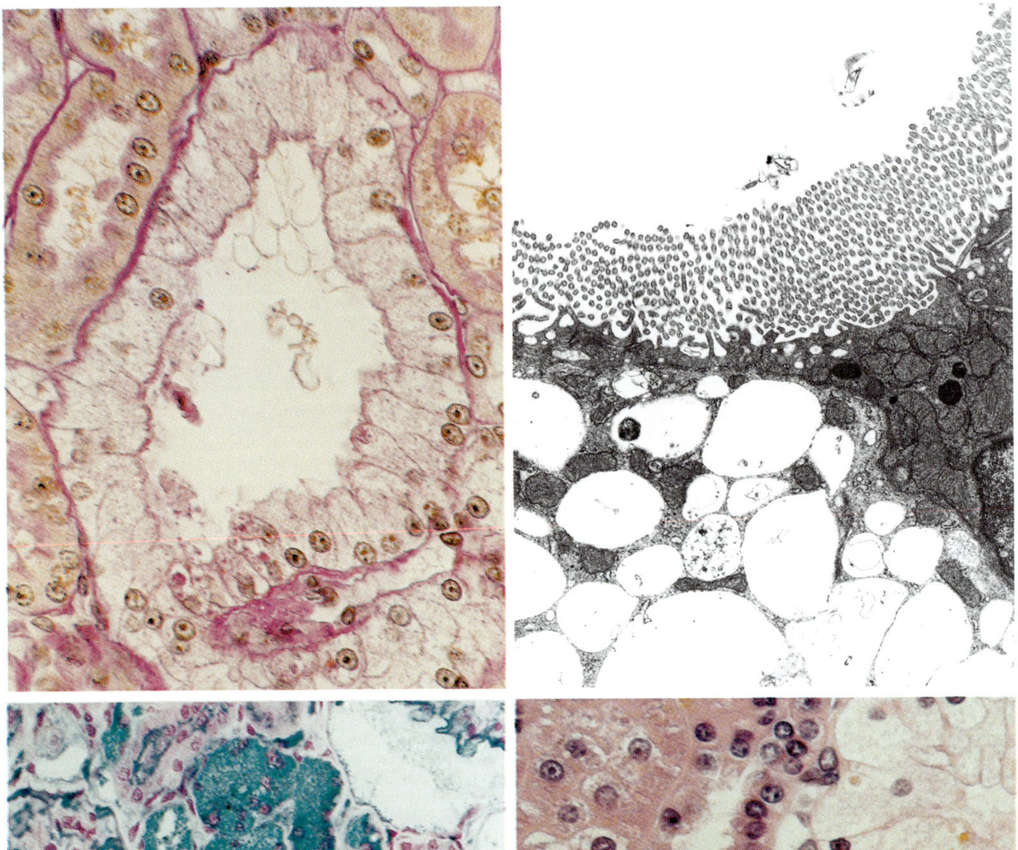

2A 2B 2C 2D

of connotations with our increasing understanding of the biological significance of the different types of altered tubules [14].

Cellular Origin and Fine Structure

Chromophobic Cell Tubules and Tumors

Chromophobic renal cell tubules and tumors (fig. 2) appear to be relatively rare and have hitherto only been described in rats exposed to some chemicals [18, 21, 35, 36] or carrying the predisposing Eker gene [9]. The site of origin of the chromophobic cells is the proximal nephron as demonstrated by light and electron microscopy [14, 21, 36]. In both altered tubules and tumors, the chromophobic cellular phenotype is characterized by unusually large polyhedral cells that contain numerous cytoplasmic vacuoles, and may show an apical brush border like normal cells of the proximal tubule. In conventional tissue sections stained with hematoxylin and eosin the chromophobic cells may be mistaken for clear glycogen storage cells at first glance, but a closer look reveals a foamy cytoplasm, which instead of glycogen may store abundant glycosaminoglycans as demonstrated by staining with alcian blue or the iron-binding reaction. Chromophobic renal cell tumors induced in rats by nitrosamines appeared as small, well-demarcated lesions, which were classified as adenomas [36, 37]. However, in rats exposed to streptozotocin, larger tumors containing both chromophobic and basophilic components developed which were classified as carcinomas [37]. The ultrastructure of renal epithelial tumors induced in mice by streptozotocin also showed some features of chromophobic renal cell tumors observed in other species, but often contained larger glycogen deposits [38]. This phenomenon has previously been observed in streptozotocin-induced basophilic rat renal cell tumors, and has been explained as a consequence of the high blood glucose levels in these animals, which suffer from diabetes due to pancreatic islet cell damage by streptozotocin [1].

Basing their views on the experimental findings in rats, Thoenes et al. [22, 23] described the chromophobic renal cell carcinoma as a pathomorphologic entity in man. However, in contrast to the chromophobic rat renal cell tumor, the human chromophobic cell carcinoma has been traced to the

Fig. 2. Chromophobic renal cell tubules induced in rats with N-nitrosomorpholine. *A* Light micrograph of chromophobic renal cell tubule. Tri-PAS. × 400. *B* Electron micrograph of portion of chromophobic cell tubule containing large cytoplasmic vacuoles and forming a brush border at the luminal plasma membrane. Lead citrate. × 8,000. *C* Chromophobic renal cell tubules excessively storing glycosaminoglycans as demonstrated by the iron-binding reaction. × 200. *D* Portion of proliferating chromophobic cell tubule. HE. × 480.

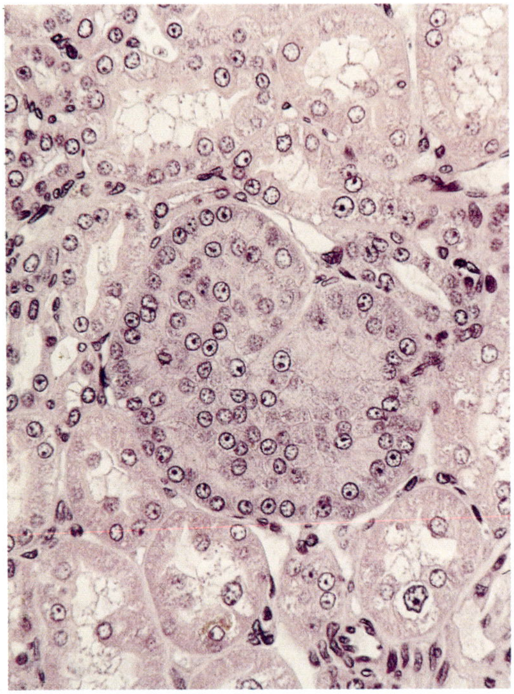

3A

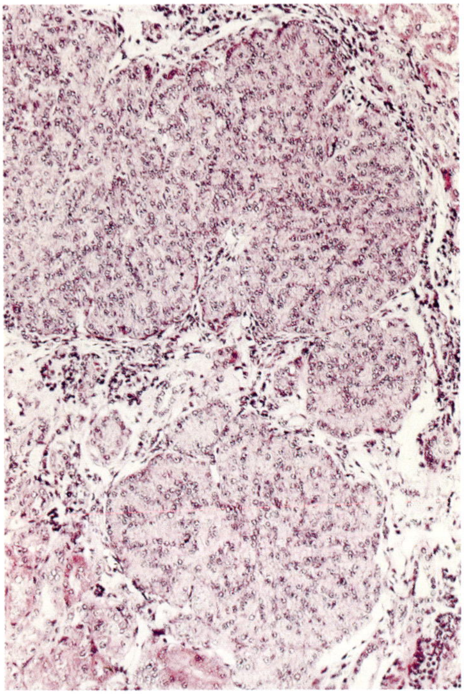

3B

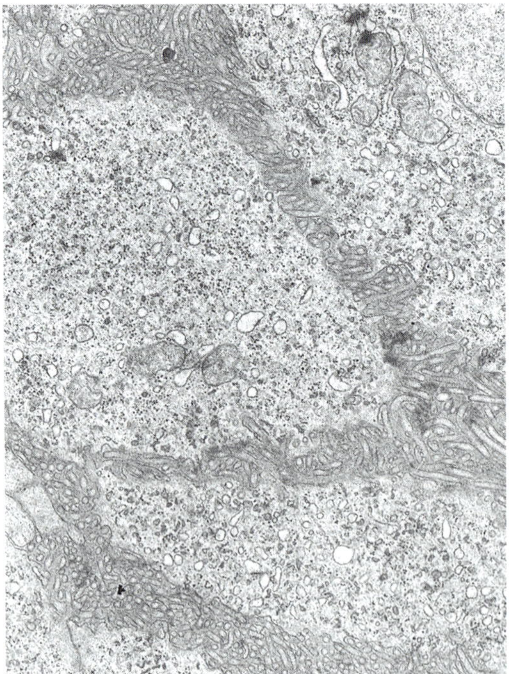

3C

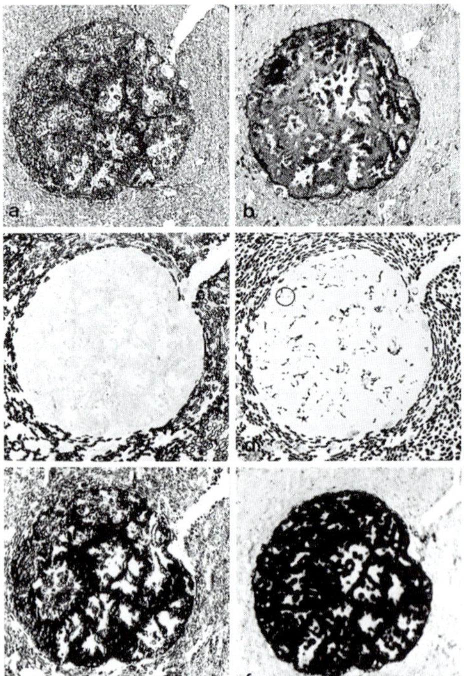

3D

collecting duct, particularly to the intercalated cells, by a histochemical approach [39, 40].

Basophilic Cell Tubules and Tumors

Basophilic cell tumors (fig. 3) are the prevailing type of renal cell tumor in rodents [11, 12, 14, 41, 42]. They may consist of small or large basophilic cells (without prominent cytoplasmic vacuoles) which form tubular, trabecular, solid, cystic or cystic-papillary structures [14]. There is general agreement that these types of tumor originate from the proximal nephron [21, 26, 27, 43–50]. Because there is frequently an intimate spatial relationship between chromophobic and basophilic cells in tubular lesions and sometimes also in tumors, we have hypothesized that the chromophobic cell lesions may represent precursors of basophilic renal cell tumors in the rat [21]. However, the relative rarity of chromophobic cell tubules as compared to basophilic cell tumors argues in favor of an origin of the majority of basophilic cell neoplasms from hyperbasophilic tubules, in line with previous notions of many authors [14, 41, 44, 45, 50].

Many of these hyperbasophilic tubules show a slight storage of glycosaminoglycans, indicating certain similarities in metabolic aberrations to those in chromophobic cell tubules [14, 21]. Different segments of the proximal nephron have been described as sites of origin of basophilic cell tumors by different carcinogens: P_3 for N-(4-fluoro-4-biphenyl)acetamide [50]; P_2 and P_3 for N-nitrosodiethylamine [36]; P_2, P_3C and P_3M for lead acetate [36], and P_1 and P_2 for sodium barbital [31].

The hyperbasophilic renal cell tubules may be composed of small or large cells [21]. The hyperbasophilic cell tubules consisting of large cells appear to be particularly prone to progress to expanded basophilic cell tumors classified as carcinomas. Cell proliferation has been shown to be significantly increased in these basophilic cell tumors (fig. 4) compared to their tissue of origin [14, 51]. The characteristic ultrastructural features of the basophilic cell tumors are abundant free and membrane-bound ribosomes, and more or less elaborate brush border formations of their plasma membrane, indicating their origin from the proximal nephron [21, 43–46]. There is little doubt that many small basophilic cell tumors represent only early stages of the larger lesions. This

Fig. 3. Basophilic renal cell lesions induced in rats with N-nitrosomorpholine. *A* Renal tubule composed of enlarged hyperbasophilic cells. HE. × 380. *B* Basophilic renal cell tumor. HE. × 120. *C* Electron micrograph of portion of basophilic cells containing abundant ribosomes and forming brush borders. Lead citrate. × 9,500. *D* Serial sections of basophilic renal cell tumor showing pronounced changes in basophilia (*a*), glycogen content (*b*), and activities of glucose-6-phosphatase (*c*), adenosinetriphosphatase (*d*), glyceraldehyde-3-phosphate dehydrogenase (*e*), and glucose-6-phosphate dehydrogenase (*f*). × 12.

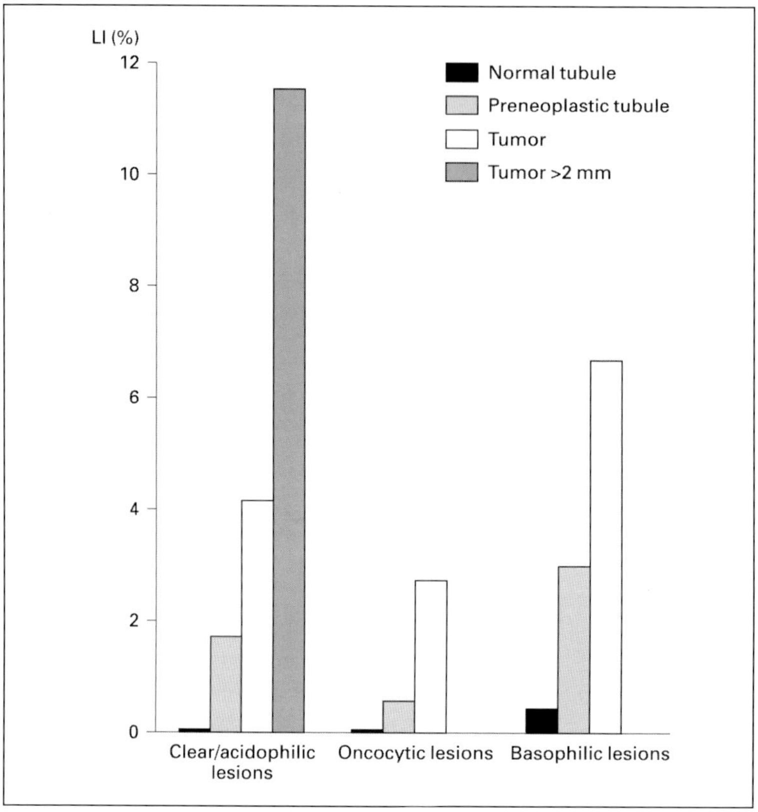

Fig. 4. Labeling index (LI) of [^{3}H]-thymidine administered continuously for 48 h in different types of N-nitrosomorpholine-induced types of rat renal cell tumors and their respective tubular site of origin. From Bannasch et al. [14].

may also be true of cystic lesions composed of large basophilic cells [14]. However, it is unlikely that cystic lesions which are made up of small basophilic cells, especially those lined by flat epithelia, also have the potential to progress to malignant stages.

Basophilic renal cell tumors which consist of unusually large basophilic cells containing prominent vacuoles have rarely been explicitly mentioned in

Fig. 5. Light micrographs of clear cells in renal tubular lesions induced in rats with N-nitrosomorpholine. *A* Cortical collecting duct partly lined by clear cells. HE. × 300. *B* Excessive storage of glycogen in renal clear cell tubule. Tri-PAS. × 190. *C* Excessive storage of glycogen in some cells of proximal renal tubule. Tri-PAS. × 470. *D* Portion of mixed clear/acidophilic (granular) cell tumor. HE. × 255.

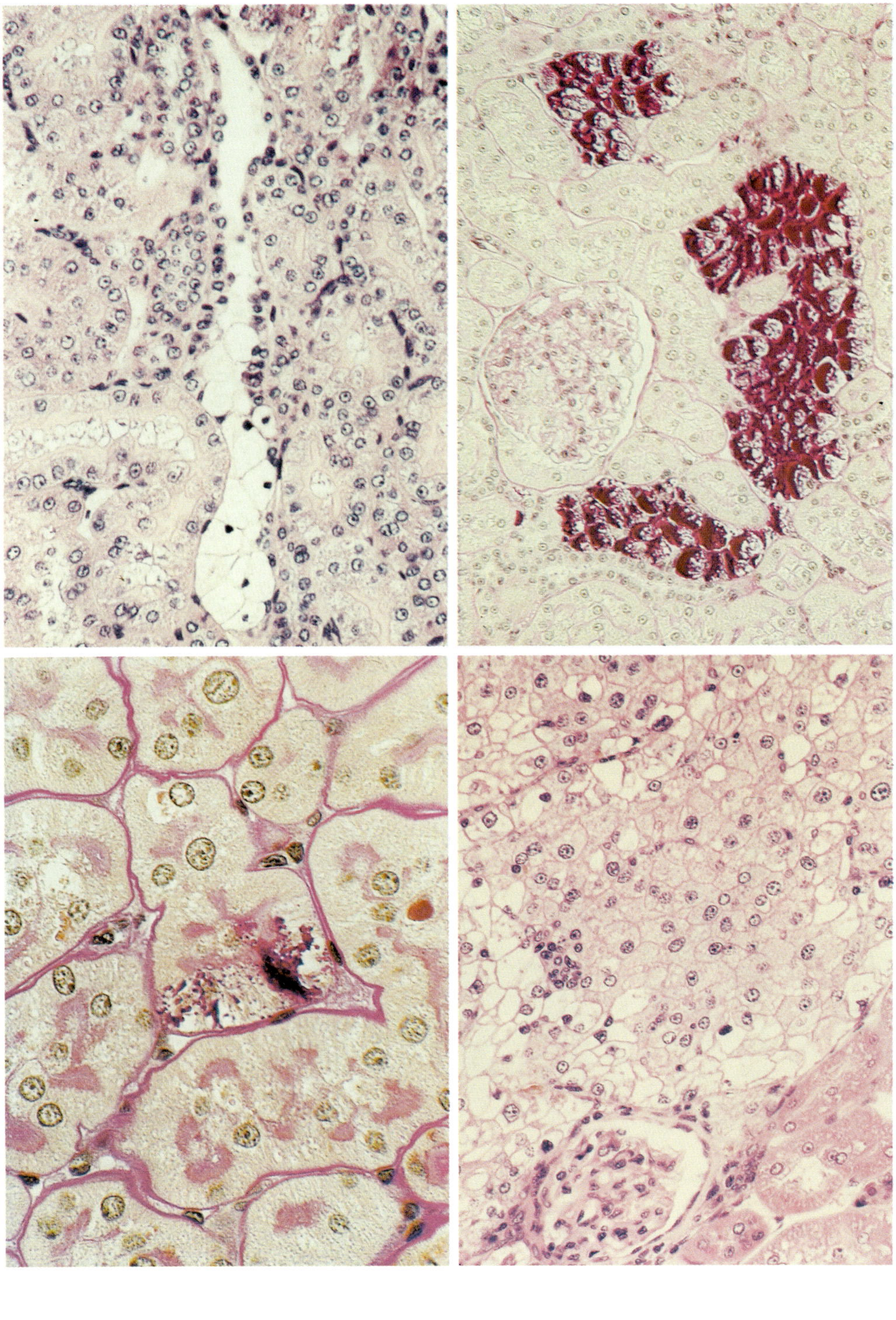

5A 5B 5C 5D

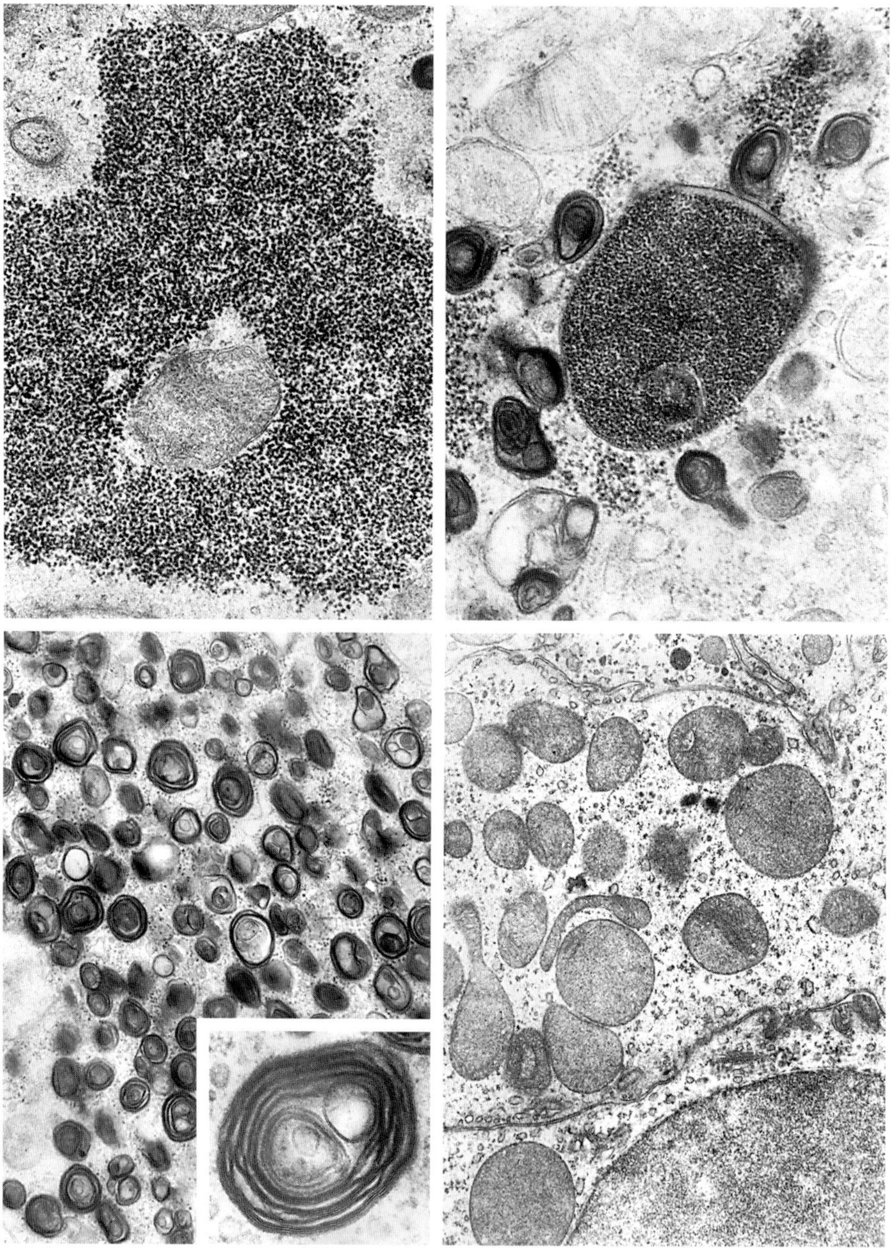

A *B* *C* *D*

Fig. 6. Electron micrographs of clear and acidophilic cells from renal cell tumors induced in rats with N-nitrosomorpholine. *A* Abundant monoparticulate glycogen in cytoplasmic matrix of clear cell. Lead citrate. × 24,000. *B* Autophagic vacuole accumulating monoparticulate glycogen. Lead citrate. × 33,000. *C* Abundant lipid bodies showing a characteristic the literature [37, 51]. In contrast to the more common basophilic cell tumors described above, this rare type of basophilic cell tumor appears to derive from the collecting duct system [52]. According to Brummer and Rabes [51], who have characterized this tumor type in some detail, it shows a clearly increased cell proliferation compared to the corresponding normal renal parenchyma.

Clear and Acidophilic (Granular) Cell Tubules and Tumors

The majority of neoplastic lesions of this type, which is not uncommon in rodents exposed to oncogenic agents and largely corresponds to the predominant type of human renal cell carcinoma, is populated by a mixture of pleomorphic clear and acidophilic cells [14, 19]. Only preneoplastic tubular lesions and small microscopic tumors may be exclusively composed of clear cells, the nuclear chromatin of which is usually highly condensed (fig. 5). In electron microscopic investigations of clear/acidophilic rat renal cell tumors, which macroscopically may become very large, the clear cells (fig. 6A–C) have been shown to contain a considerable amount of monoparticulate glycogen (localized within the cytoplasmic matrix or enclosed in autophagic vacuoles) and/or characteristic lipid bodies, the fine structure of which suggests their composition of gangliosides [14, 19]. In contrast, the cytoplasm of the acidophilic cells is poor in both glycogen and lipids, but often contains abundant mitochondria poor in cristae (fig. 6D), which are most probably responsible for the frequent granular appearance of this cell type at the light microscopic level. Intermediate clear-acidophilic cellular phenotypes are regularly intermingled between the more distinct clear and acidophilic cell populations. The characteristic lipid bodies found in rat renal clear cell tumors were subsequently also described in human renal clear cell carcinomas [53], but here the lipids usually appear as neutral lipid droplets.

The development of clear cell tumors and of mixed clear/acidophilic cell tumors from the clear cell tubules excessively storing glycogen has been established by cytomorphological, cytochemical, and stereological approaches [19, 27, 54, 55]. In serial sections of a total of 93 clear cell-containing renal lesions induced in rats with N-nitrosomorpholine, these clear cell tubules have been shown to be usually directly connected with the collecting duct system, but not with any other part of the tubular system [54]. The preferential origin of the clear cell tubules from the collecting duct has been supported by histochemical studies [51, 55]. In recent stereological reconstructions of serial sections from 9 rat renal clear cell lesions produced by N-ethyl-N-hydroxyethylnitrosamine, 4 of 9 lesions each were found to be connected with the collecting

pattern of dark and light lines (inset, × 56,000) in clear cell. Lead citrate. × 13,500. *D* Abundant mitochondria poor in cristae in acidophilic cell. Lead citrate. × 12,800.

duct system and the distal tubule, but 1 of 9 lesions showed continuity with the proximal tubule [27]. Occasionally, small groups of clear cells were previously noted in the proximal nephron (fig. 5C) of carcinogen-treated rats [19, 54], but clear cell tumors deriving from this part of the nephron had not been unequivocally demonstrated. In contrast to the experimental findings, the human clear and granular cell carcinomas are considered to originate from the proximal nephron by most authors [24, 25, 56], as suggested years ago by the electron microscopic findings of Oberling et al. [57], although distal parts of the renal tubular system, including the collecting duct, have been discussed as the possible site of origin of these tumor types in humans as well [54, 58].

Many observations endorse the notion that the mixed clear/acidophilic (granular) cell tumors arise from clear cell tubules or small clear cell tumors (adenomas) in which the cells gradually lose their glycogen and progress to a more malignant state [14, 19, 27, 51, 55]. In clear cell tubules and adenomas, DNA synthesis as determined by [^{3}H]thymidine incorporation (fig. 4) is only slightly increased [14], but a marked elevation in the labeling index takes place when large clear/acidophilic cell tumors develop [14, 51], justifying their classification as carcinomas. During conversion from clear to acidophilic cells, the initially highly condensed nuclear chromatin undergoes a striking decondensation [19]. Additional support for an interconversion between clear and granular cells during neoplastic development comes from recent investigations on mutations in the von Hippel-Lindau (VHL) gene in clear/granular cell tumors induced in rats with N-nitrosodiethylamine [59]. Three of the 8 clear cell-containing tumors studied showed mutations of the rat VHL gene, which were uniform in the mixed clear/granular cell populations in 2 cases. In human patients suffering from tuberous sclerosis or VHL disease, who are at high risk of developing renal clear/granular cell carcinomas, atypical cysts lined by clear cells like experimentally induced tubular or cystic lesions have been described to be associated with the carcinomas [60], suggesting striking interspecies similarities in the cellular evolution of this tumor type.

Oncocytic Tubules and Oncocytomas

This type of renal cell tumor frequently develops in the rat exposed to chemical carcinogens, but may also occur 'spontaneously' in old animals [5, 13, 18, 20, 27, 49, 61]. The renal oncocytoma has been known for some time from human pathology [62], but only attracted greater attention when several reports provided evidence for a more frequent occurrence and benign behavior [23, 24, 63]. The oncocyte is a unique cell type defined many years ago by Hamperl [62] and well known to form neoplasms at different sites in man [62, 64].

The rat renal oncocytoma (fig. 7) is composed of large polygonal cells with an intensely acidophilic and finely granular cytoplasm [13, 20]. The fine structure of these oncocytes is most characteristic (fig. 7C): the cytoplasm is crowded with atypical mitochondria that exhibit abundant, unusually long and densely packed cristae [65]. Sometimes, the severely altered mitochondria form whorled structures or they display an intramitochondrial accumulation of glycogen.

The histogenesis of rat renal oncocytoma has been studied in detail in different models of experimental chemical carcinogenesis [5, 20, 27, 36, 61, 66]. Regardless of the carcinogenic compound used, an oncocytic transformation of epithelia of the collecting duct system (fig. 7A) was observed as the initial event. In addition, it was established that these neoplasms derive from both principal and intercalated cells lining the cortical and outer medullary portions of the collecting duct system [61]. In addition to oncocytes, clear cells excessively storing glycogen (fig. 7B) were rarely found in the same tubular segments (which are also the site of origin of clear cell tumors in the rat), but their possible involvement in the genesis of oncocytomas remains obscure [20, 54]. As a rule, the oncocytic tubules and oncocytomas develop in a multicentric fashion in both kidneys, and they are frequently combined with other types of tubular lesions and epithelial kidney tumors [1].

The rat renal oncocytoma grows very slowly and appears to be a benign end-stage lesion which does not progress to a malignant tumor [13]. This view is substantiated by the observation that DNA synthesis as demonstrated by the incorporation of [^{3}H]thymidine (fig. 4) is significantly increased in oncocytomas compared to the normal cortical collecting duct, but it is much less elevated than in basophilic and clear/acidophilic renal cell tumors.

There is general agreement that the human renal oncocytoma originates from the collecting duct system like the rat renal oncocytoma [39, 67, 68]. However, results of immunohistochemical studies favored their origin from intercalated rather than principal cells of the collecting duct [39]. Moreover, on the basis of lectin-binding studies, Eble and Hull [69] suggest that even the possibility of a proximal tubular origin [70] has to be reconsidered for some human renal oncocytomas.

Mechanisms of Neoplastic Cell Conversion

Toxicity and Hyperplasia

Various nonspecific toxic effects have been implicated in the mechanism of renal carcinogenesis. At the tissue level, a hyperplastic response to toxic cell necrosis has been regarded as an early event in renal carcinogenesis by

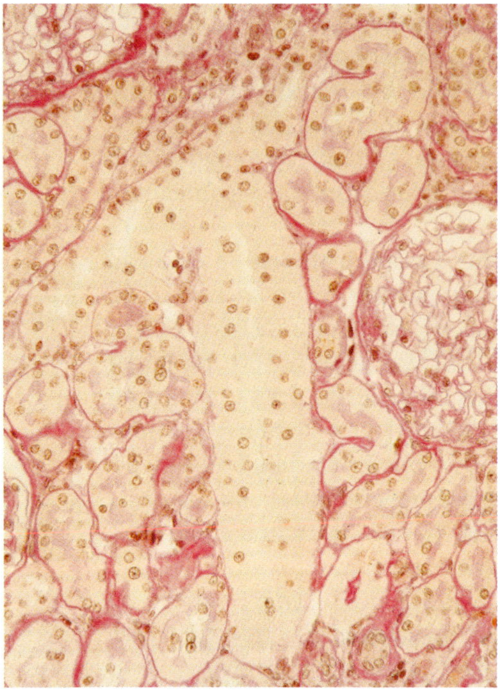

7A

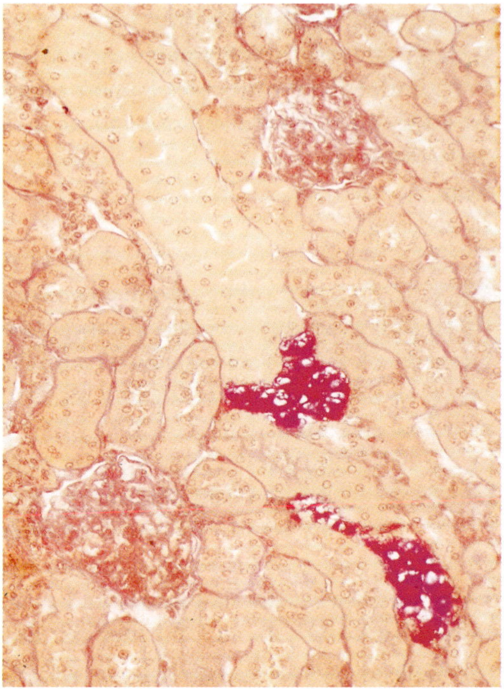

7B

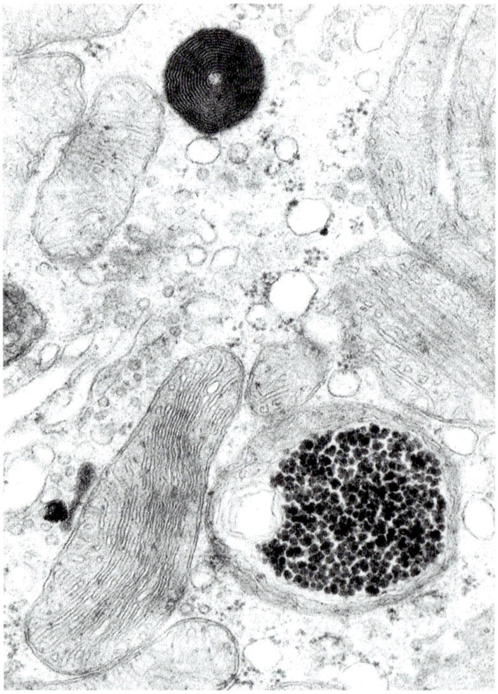

7C

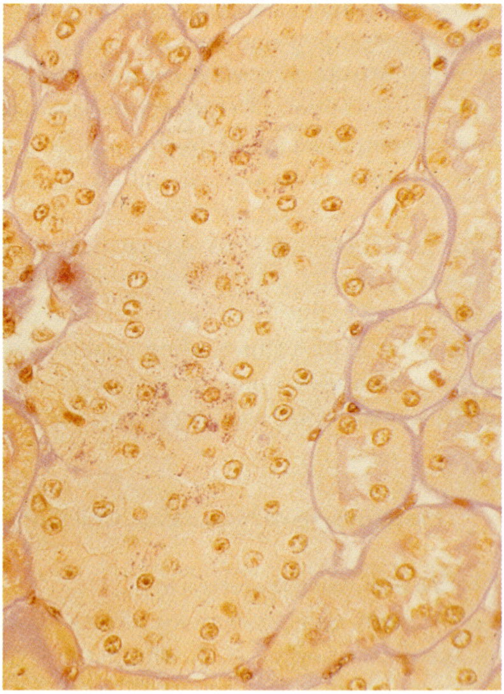

7D

many authors [11, 12, 30, 41, 45, 71–76]. Hyperplasia elicited by nonspecific toxic lesions has been discussed in particular as a possible cause of neoplastic renal cell conversion when the carcinogenic agent did not show mutagenic activity in a number of in vitro assays [11, 12, 30]. A well-known representative of this group of agents is the cationic chelator nitrilotriacetic acid, which is toxic to the epithelial cells of the proximal tubule and leads to cytoplasmic vacuolation and occasional cell necrosis [77, 78]. Anderson et al. [79] suggested that the toxic effect of nitrilotriacetic acid might be associated with a divalent cation imbalance resulting in increased levels of divalent cations, such as Zn^+ and Ca^+, providing a constant stimulus for cell proliferation.

Several important industrial and environmental chemicals, including volatile hydrocarbons, have been shown to produce an intralysosomal accumulation of the urinary protein α_{2n}-globulin in epithelial cells of the proximal tubule and eventually exert toxic effects leading to cell death in male rats [11, 30, 33, 80]. In case of continuous exposure to such compounds, the cellular necrosis elicits a sustained elevation of cell proliferation which is considered to be related to the formation of preneoplastic and neoplastic renal lesions.

Karyocytomegaly has also been linked with neoplastic renal cell conversion, but several authors agree that this alteration is most likely a result of toxic damage and is not a reliable indicator of a carcinogenic response [45, 50, 76].

The frequent origin of rat renal cell tumors from the collecting duct system is hardly compatible with the notion of an initiating regenerative hyperplastic stimulus by toxic cell necrosis, which predominantly occurs in the proximal nephron [14]. The results of stop experiments with N-nitrosomorpholine in rats likewise jeopardize the suggested significance of tubular necrosis and hyperplasia in the evolution of epithelial renal neoplasms [1]. With the exception of very high sublethal doses [81], neither early necrotic nor hyperplastic changes were observed during the period of carcinogen exposure. The majority of preneoplastic tubular lesions preceding the manifestation of neoplasms emerged weeks and months after withdrawal of the carcinogenic agent [14–21]. While no increase in cell proliferation was detected by autoradiographic determination of the incorporation of [^{3}H]-thymidine during the period of carcino-

Fig. 7. Oncocytic tubules and oncocytoma induced in rats with N-nitrosomorpholine. *A* Light micrograph of oncocytic tubule connected with cortical collecting duct. Tri-PAS. × 240. *B* Light micrograph of oncocytic tubule containing some cells excessively storing glycogen. Tri-PAS. × 180. *C* Electron micrograph of portion of oncocyte showing abundant mitochondria containing densely packed cristae and sometimes glycogen. Lead citrate. × 32,500. *D* Light micrograph of small oncocytoma containing some glycogen particles. Tri-PAS. × 330.

gen administration [1], there was an ever-increasing cell proliferation from the preneoplastic tubular lesions through small-to-large neoplasms [14, 51].

Metabolic Cellular Changes and Growth Factors

Investigations on different types of human renal cell tumor suggested to some authors that the diversity in cellular phenotypes may not indicate an origin from special segments of the tubular system, but might reflect an abnormal gene expression associated with neoplastic changes in certain cell clones [82], or result from several options for differentiation of a common precursor stem cell [83]. Although there is, undoubtedly, a great plasticity in the neoplastic phenotype of renal cell tumors, the consistent appearance of cytologically well-defined tumor types, the origin of which has been traced to certain cell types of the renal tubular system which undergo characteristic metabolic changes as demonstrated by cytochemical and biochemical approaches, indicates ordered sequential events in several cell lineages leading to the different types of renal cell tumors [1]. Fundamental changes in energy metabolism have been detected during the evolution of all types of renal cell tumor and, hence, seem to be a common denominator of neoplastic renal cell conversion [14, 26, 84]. The variations in phenotypic expression of renal cell tumors may mainly depend on the specific state of differentiation of the respective cells of origin. The nature of the oncogenic agent may also have some influence. However, from a review on preneoplastic lesions in the rodent kidney, it appears that genotoxic and nongenotoxic chemicals produce in principal the same types of lesion [30]. This also holds true for animals carrying a predisposing gene as demonstrated for the hereditary Eker rat renal cell tumors [9].

The most striking early phenotypic cellular changes indicating metabolic aberrations during the development of renal cell tumors are an excessive storage of glycogen (glycogenosis) or glycosaminoglycans (mucopolysaccharidosis) in clear and chromophobic/basophilic cells, respectively, and an accumulation of abnormal mitochondria in oncocytes (oncocytosis) [26]. As described in some detail above, the glycogenotic clear cells are gradually transformed into acidophilic cells during progression from preneoplastic tubular lesions to advanced neoplasms [19]. Enzyme and immunohistochemical studies on the glycogenotic clear cell tubules and clear/acidophilic cell tumors have shown that in comparison to the normal epithelium of the collecting duct (from which the majority of these lesions develop) the glycogenotic tubules have an increased activity of glycogen phosphorylase and reduced activities in several glycolytic enzymes (e.g. hexokinase, glyceraldehyde-3-phosphate dehydrogenase, pyruvate kinase) and mitochondrial enzymes (e.g. succinate dehydrogenase), accompanied by a strongly reduced expression of the glucose transporter, GLUT1 [55]. Moderately increased activities of glycolytic and mitochondrial enzymes, and of the key enzyme of the pentose phosphate pathway, glucose-6-phosphate dehydrogenase, were observed in clear/acidophilic cell tubules and tumors compared with those in glycogenotic tubules. These findings suggest that glycogen storage is not due to an increased uptake of glucose from the blood, but results from a disturbance in the intracellular flux of metabolites. The enzymatic alterations during the emergence of glycogenotic clear cells from the collecting duct epithelium, and their conversion into glycogen-poor acidophilic cells during progression indicate a fundamental shift in energy metabolism which is closely linked to the process of neoplastic cell transformation [55, 84].

Enzyme histochemical investigations in human clear cell carcinomas (which are considered to originate from the proximal nephron) revealed metabolic aberrations similar to those observed in rat renal cell tumors [84]. This applies especially to a decreased activity of the glucose-6-phosphatase and increased activity of the glyceraldehyde-3-phosphate dehydrogenase, suggesting a high glycolysis at the expense of gluconeogenesis. The histochemical results largely agree with biochemical findings [85–87]. In addition to the enzymatic alterations, the biochemical studies provided evidence for an increased level of glucose-6-phosphate [86, 87]. The primary biochemical lesion leading to these metabolic alterations remains obscure, but there are many similarities with sequential metabolic aberrations in experimental and human hepatocarcinogenesis, which appear to result from early alterations in intracellular signal transduction as discussed in some detail elsewhere [88–90]. This holds particularly true for renal clear cell lesions excessively storing glycogen and/or lipids and the metabolic aberrations mimicking insulin effects in glycogenotic preneoplastic or early neoplastic hepatocellular lesions. Increased activities of the insulin- and insulin-like growth factor-I receptor tyrosine kinase [91] and an overexpression of the mitogen-activated protein kinase, which are involved in the insulin-stimulated signal transduction pathway, have actually been reported to occur in human renal cell carcinomas [92].

Comparable metabolic changes might be related to the genesis of chromophobic and basophilic renal cell tumors, although the early events are poorly understood in this case. The tumors arise from chromophobic and basophilic cells in tubules frequently accumulating glycosaminoglycans [21]. Tumor progression is usually associated with a gradual loss of these polysaccharides. Enzyme histochemical studies in basophilic rat renal cell tumors suggested that a marked shift of energy metabolism from oxidative to glycolytic production of ATP with a corresponding reduction in mitochondrial respiration is characteristic of this tumor type [66, 84, 93]. The preneoplastic basophilic cell tubules induced in the rat kidney with nitrosamines or streptozotocin share a number of metabolic aberrations (as detected by cytochemical methods) with the basophilic renal cell tumors; however, some intriguing differences are also noteworthy [14]. These tubular lesions and very small basophilic renal cell tumors already show a loss in the activities of the mitochondrial enzyme succinate dehydrogenase [66], the microsomal glucose-6-phosphatase [66], and the membrane bound enzyme γ-glutamyltranspeptidase [66, 94, 95] and a reduced expression of the glucose transporter GLUT2 [96], while the activities of the glycolytic enzymes hexokinase and pyruvate kinase are elevated [96]. In addition, markedly increased binding of antibodies to glutathione S-transferase A and elevated levels of four cytochrome P-450 species and the microsomal epoxide hydrolase have been observed in the majority of basophilic tubules immunohistochemically [95, 97]. Whereas binding to two of the cytochromes and to glucose-6-phosphate dehydrogenase tended to be even greater in larger, more advanced lesions, a late decrease in binding to epoxide hydrolase and glutathione S-transferase A was evident. The activities of glucose-6-phosphate dehydrogenase and glyceralde-3-phosphate dehydrogenase were usually increased in both basophilic tubules and tumors [66]. Because the pentose phosphate shunt, among other functions, also provides pentoses for RNA and DNA synthesis, activation of this pathway is probably closely related to the increase in ribosomes and enhanced cellular proliferation in the basophilic preneoplastic and neoplastic lesions [1].

The oncocytic tubules and tumors differ in their histochemical pattern from both the chromophobic/basophilic and the clear/acidophilic renal cell lesions [66, 84]. Detailed enzyme and immunohistochemical studies on rat renal oncocytic lesions revealed that the activities of several enzymes of glucose metabolism (e.g. glucose-6-phosphatase, glycogen synthase, glycogen phosphorylase, glyceraldehyde-3-phosphate dehydrogenase) and the expression of the glucose transporter, GLUT2, were similar to those of the normal collecting duct, whereas the activities and/or content of mitochondrial enzymes (succinate dehydrogenase, cytochrome-c-oxidase) and glycolytic enzymes (hexokinase, pyruvate kinase) and the expression of the glucose transporter GLUT1 were markedly increased in oncocytomas compared to the collecting duct system [97–99]. Of particular interest is that, in contrast to other types of rat renal cell tumors, the activity of the rate-limiting enzyme of the pentose phosphate pathway, glucose-6-phosphate dehydrogenase, is normal or even decreased in oncocytomas, suggesting that a relatively low supply of precursors for the synthesis of nucleic acids and phospholipids might be responsible for the slow growth of this tumor type [1, 66]. A specific metabolic mitochondrial defect which might explain the abundance of mitochondria in oncocytes as a result of a compensatory hyperplasia, in line with suggestions by a number of authors [100, 101], has hitherto not been identified. It is conceivable, however, that the metabolic changes associated with the accumulation of the mitochondria play a decisive role in the development of the most characteristic neoplastic phenotype of the renal oncocyte.

Expression of the tumor growth factor-α (TGFα), which is limited to the collecting ducts and to the proximal tubules under normal conditions, was found in the hereditary renal cell carcinoma of the Eker rat [102]. TGFα has also been shown to be expressed in regenerative proximal tubular epithelium and in renal cell carcinomas induced in rats by ferric nitrilotriacetate [103].

Molecular Genetic Changes

In contrast to the extensive investigations on chromosomal aberrations and molecular genetic changes in human renal cell carcinomas [104], only a few studies on molecular genetic changes in renal carcinogenesis induced by chemicals in rodents have been conducted [15]. The genotoxic carcinogen dimethylnitrosamine has been shown to interact with DNA in the rat kidney and to produce two major DNA adducts, namely N^7-methylguanine and O^6-methylguanine [105]. Whereas N^7-methylguanine is rapidly removed from renal tissue by repair processes, O^6-methylguanine persists over longer time periods and may represent a promutagenic lesion [106]. Some renal carcinogens are apparently not directly genotoxic but might lead to DNA damage by indirect mechanisms. Thus, it has been discussed that ferric nitriloacetate might exert its carcinogenic effect through DNA damage [107, 108] induced by oxygen radicals [109], as suggested by increased levels of 8-hydroxydeoxyguanosine (8-OH-dG) that is regarded as a marker of oxidative DNA damage. Free radical-induced lipid peroxidation, as indicated by the formation of 4-hydroxy-2-nonenal, has also been demonstrated in the rat kidney exposed to ferric nitriloacetate [110]. In addition, potassium bromate, which produces a high incidence of renal cell tumors in rats without being directly genotoxic, has been shown to increase lipid peroxidation [111] and the level of 8-OH-dG [112] in the kidney.

Mutations in the VHL gene were frequently found in human renal cell carcinomas, particularly in clear cell carcinomas [113]. Several groups failed to detect similar mutations in chemically induced or spontaneous rat renal cell tumors or tumor cell lines [114–116] of various phenotypes. However, clear cell tumors and mixed clear/acidophilic cell tumors induced in rats by N-nitrosodimethylamine were only recently screened for such mutations [59]. Three of the eight renal cell tumors studied showed four (three G:C to A:T and one A:T to G:C) mutations of the VHL gene, suggesting that the rat renal clear and clear/acidophilic cell tumor may be an appropriate model of changes in both the genotype and the phenotype of the predominant type of human renal cell carcinoma.

Matsumoto et al. [117] reported the absence of point mutations at several codons of ras family genes in rat renal cell tumors induced by N-ethyl-N-hydroxyethylnitrosamine and N-nitrosomorpholine.

In the past few years hereditary renal cell carcinoma of the rat [6] has been extensively investigated as a model of a Mendelian dominantly inherited cancer [9, 10]. Chromophilic (basophilic and eosinophilic) [118], chromophobic [119], and 'oncocyte-like' cells [120] that most probably correspond to the chromophilic variant, but no clear/acidophilic (granular) cell phenotypes were described in this hereditary renal cell carcinoma. Exposure of adult Eker rats to N-nitrosodimethylamine [121] and ionizing radiation [119] considerably increased the incidence of renal cell adenomas and carcinomas. The Eker rat has also been shown to be highly susceptible to the induction of renal cell tumors by transplacental administration of ethylnitrosourea [119]. The predisposing gene of the Eker rat was mapped to chromosome 10 [119, 122, 123] and identified as a germline mutation in the rat homologue of the human tuberous sclerosis gene (Tsc2) [122, 124].

Loss of heterozygosity (LOH) of the wild-type Tsc2 allele was demonstrated in approximately 60% of spontaneous renal cell tumors in the Eker rat [125]. Along with the observation that the induction of large adenomas and carcinomas in the Eker rat by ionizing radiation follows a linear dose-response [119], LOH at chromosome 10 indicated that in heterozygotes two events (one inherited, one somatic) are necessary for tumor production [125]. Using laser microdissection, Kubo et al. [126] have shown that LOH of the wild-type Tsc2 gene occurs even in 21% of preneoplastic, phenotypically altered tubules, supporting the hypothesis that a second somatic mutation is a rate-limiting step for renal carcinogenesis in the Eker rat, as well as suggesting a tumor-suppressor function of the Tsc2 gene. Additional support for this hypothesis has been provided by the finding that wild-type Tsc2 gene transfer into cell lines derived from Eker renal cell tumors suppresses the neoplastic phenotype [127, 128]. In a transgenic Eker rat with a wild-type Tsc2 gene, Kobayashi et al. [129] verified that germline suppression of the Eker phenotype is possible for both embryonic lethality of the homozygote and tumor predisposition in the heterozygote.

Approximately 40% of spontaneous and ethylnitrosourea-induced renal cell tumors in the Eker rat retain the wild-type Tsc2 allele [119, 125]. The presence of intragenic Tsc2 somatic mutations in LOH-negative renal cell tumors, which were qualitatively different in spontaneous and chemically induced tumors, has been demonstrated in 33% of the 30 tumors studied [130]. These subtle mutations or epigenetic mechanisms may result in an inactivation of the Tsc2 gene in the absence of LOH. Recently, a high frequency of somatic mutations in the Tsc2 gene, which was biallelic in some cases, was found in renal cell tumors induced in non-Eker rats by N-ethyl-N-hydroxyethylnitrosamine or N-nitrosodimethylamine [131, 132].

The functions of the Tsc2 product called 'tuberin' are not fully understood, but it has been reported that it has weak GTPase-activating protein activity for Rap 1a [133] and Rab 5 [134], possesses potential transcriptional activation domains (AD1 and AD2) [135], and might contribute to the regulation of the cell cycle and cell survival [136].

Conclusions

Animal models of renal cell adenomas and carcinomas in rodents, particularly in rats, have been shown to be very valuable for the elucidation of the pathogenesis of the most prevalent types of human kidney tumors. Chemically induced rat renal cell tumors proved to be an excellent tool for separating different tumor types by cytomorphological and simple cytochemical criteria. The classification of rat renal cell tumors based on these findings has been adopted in a modified form for human pathology. The cellular origin and the sequence of cellular changes during the development of the different types of rat renal cell tumors has been largely clarified. In addition to the proximal nephron, the collecting duct system was first identified as a frequent site of origin of renal cell tumors in the experimental models. It has rapidly been shown that this also holds true for human epithelial kidney tumors, although some discrepancies between the experimental findings and the observations in human pathology are evident in this respect.

The sequential changes in the cellular phenotypes during rat renal carcinogenesis indicated a fundamental shift in energy metabolism during neoplastic cell conversion in all types of tumor, suggesting early disturbances in signal transduction pathways, which may result in characteristic metabolic responses in each of the specifically differentiated cell types along the renal tubular system. This knowledge remains to be fully exploited for our understanding of the pathogenesis of human renal cell tumors.

Mutations of the VHL gene comparable to those known from human clear/granular cell carcinomas have recently been demonstrated to occur in clear/granular cell carcinomas chemically induced in rats, suggesting that this animal model may be appropriate for analyzing changes in both the genotype and the phenotype of this predominant type of human renal cell carcinoma. Particularly promising progress has been made in the past 2 years in establishing the hereditary renal cell carcinoma of the Eker rat as a model of a Mendelian dominantly inherited kidney cancer, which will also help to understand the interaction of genetic and environmental factors in the evolution or renal cell tumors.

References

1 Bannasch P, Zerban H: Animal models and renal carcinogenesis; in Eble JN (ed): Tumors and Tumor-Like Conditions of the Kidneys and Ureters. New York, Churchill Livingstone, 1990, pp 1–34.

2 Hard GC: Tumors of the kidney, renal pelvis and ureter; in Turusov VS, Mohr U (eds): Pathology of Tumours in Laboratory Animals, vol I. Tumours of the Rat, part II, ed 2. Lyon, International Agency for Research in Cancer, 1990, pp 301–344.

3 Hiasa Y, Ito N: Experimental induction of renal tumors. Crit Rev Toxicol 1987;17:279–343.

4 Jones TC, Hard GC, Mohr U (eds): Urinary System, ed 2. Berlin, Springer, 1997.

5 Nogueira E, Cardesa A, Mohr U: Experimental models of kidney tumors. J Cancer Res Clin Oncol 1993;119:190–198.

6 Eker R: Familial renal adenomas in Wistar rats. A preliminary report. Acta Pathol Microbiol Scand 1954;34:554–562.

7 Eker R, Mossige JA: A dominant gene for renal adenomas in the rats. Nature 1961;189:858–859.

8 Everitt JL, Goldsworthy TL, Wolf DC, Walker CL: Hereditary renal cell carcinoma in the Eker rat: A unique animal model for the study of cancer susceptibility. Toxicol Lett 1996;82:621–625.

9 Hino O, Mitani H, Kobayashi T, Tsuchiya H, Orimoto K, Kikuchi Y, Urakami S, Yamamoto T, Kajino K: Pathophysiological features of hereditary cancers. Gann Monogr Cancer Res 1996;44:175–187.

10 Everitt JI, Walker CL, Goldsworthy T, Wolf DC: Hereditary renal cell adenoma and carcinoma, rat; in Jones TC, Hard GC, Mohr U (eds): Urinary System, ed 2. Berlin, Springer, 1997, pp 173–179.

11 Lipsky MM Jr, Trump BF: Chemically induced renal epithelial neoplasia in experimental animals. Int Rev Exp Pathol 1988;30:357–383.

12 Konishi N, Hiasa Y: Renal carcinogenesis; in Waalkes MP, Ward JM (eds): Carcinogenesis, New York, Raven Press, 1994, pp 123–159.

13 Bannasch P, Zerban H, Ahn YS, Hacker HJ: Oncocytoma, kidney, rat; in Jones TC, Hard GC, Mohr U (eds): Urinary System, ed 2. Berlin, Springer, 1997, pp 64–79.

14 Bannasch P, Zerban H, Ahn US, Hacker HJ: Renal cell adenoma and carcinoma, kidney, rat; in Jones TC, Hard GC, Mohr U (eds): Urinary System, ed 2. Berlin, Springer, 1997, pp 79–118.

15 Hard GC: Renal carcinogenesis, rat; in Jones TC, Hard GC, Mohr U (eds): Urinary System, ed 2. Berlin, Springer, 1997, pp 58–63.

16 Boorman GA, McDonald MR, Imoto S, Persing R: Renal lesions induced by ochratoxin A exposure in the F344 rat. Toxicol Pathol 1992;20:236–245.

17 Hard GC: High frequency, single-dose model of renal adenoma/carcinoma induction using dimethylnitrosamine in Crl: (W) BR rats. Carcinogenesis 1984;5:1047–1050.

18 Bannasch P, Schacht U, Storch E: Morphogenese und Mikromorphologie epithelialer Tumoren der Niere von N-Nitrosomorpholin-vergifteten Ratten. I. Induktion und Histologie. Z Krebsforsch 1974;81:311–331.

19 Bannasch P, Krech R, Zerban H: Morphogenese und Mikromorphologie epithelialer Nierentumoren bei Nitrosomorpholin-vergifteten Ratten. II. Tubuläre Glykogenose und die Genese von klar-oder acidophilzelligen Tumoren. Z Krebsforsch 1978;92:63–86.

20 Bannasch P, Krech R, Zerban H: Morphogenese und Mikromorphologie epithelialer Nierentumoren bei Nitrosomorpholin-vergifteten Ratten. III. Onkocytentubuli und Onkocytome. Z Krebsforsch 1978;92:87–104.

21 Bannasch P, Krech R, Zerban H: Morphogenese und Mikromorphologie epithelialer Nierentumoren bei Nitrosomorpholin-vergifteten Ratten. IV. Tubuläre Läsionen und basophile Tumoren. J Cancer Res Clin Oncol 1980;98:243–265.

22 Thoenes W, Störkel S, Rumpelt HJ: Human chromophobe cell renal carcinoma. Virchows Arch B Cell Pathol 1985;48:207–217.

23 Thoenes W, Störkel S, Rumpelt HJ: Histopathology and classification of renal cell tumors (adenomas, oncocytomas, and carcinomas). The basic cytological and histopathological elements and their use for diagnostics. Pathol Res Pract 1986;181:125–143.

24 Störkel S: Karzinome und Onkozytome der Niere. Stuttgart, Fischer, 1993.

25 Murphy WM, Reckwith JB, Farrow GM: Tumors of the Kidney, Bladder, and Related Urinary Structures. Atlas of Pathology. Washington, Armed Forces Institute of Pathology, 1994.

26 Bannasch P: Sequential cellular changes during chemical carcinogenesis. J Cancer Res Clin Oncol 1984;108:11–22.
27 Tsuda H, Iwase T, Matsumoto K, Ito M, Hirono I, Nishida Y, Takasuka N, Iwahori Y, Ota T, Kim DJ, Kadenbach B: Histogenetic stereological reconstruction of rat basophilic, clear, and oncocytic neoplastic renal cell lesions using carbonic anhydrase type II-PAS double-stained sections. Toxicol Pathol 1998;26:769–776.
28 Bachmann S, Kriz W: Anatomy, cytology, ultrastructure. Nephron and collecting duct in the kidney, rat; in Jones TC, Hard GC, Mohr U (eds): Urinary System, ed 2. Berlin, 1997, pp 3–36.
29 Bannasch P, Nogueira E, Zerban H, Beck K, Mayer D: Sequential phenotypic conversion of renal epithelial cells during neoplastic development; in Feo F, Pani P, Columbano A, Garcea R (eds): Chemical Carcinogenesis. New York, Plenum Press, 1988, pp 209–216.
30 Dietrich DR, Swenberg JA: Preneoplastic lesions in rodent kidney induced spontaneously or by non-genotoxic agents: Predictive nature and comparison to lesions induced by genotoxic carcinogens. Mutat Res 1991;248:239–260.
31 Kurata Y, Diwan BA, Uno H, Rice JM, Ward JM: Pathology of preneoplastic and neoplastic renal tubular lesions induced in rats by sodium barbital, a nongenotoxic renal carcinogen and nephrotoxin. Toxicol Pathol 1993;21:35–45.
32 Riopelle JL, Jasmin G: Discussion sur la nature des tumeurs rénales induites chez le rat par le diméthylnitrosamine. Rev Can Biol 1963;22:365–381.
33 Short BG, Burnett VL, Swenberg JA: Histopathology and cell proliferation induced by 2,2,4-trimethylpentane in the male rat kidney. Toxicol Pathol 1986;14:194–203.
34 Hard GC, Alden CL, Stula EF, Trump BF: Proliferative lesions of the kidney in rats; in Guides for Toxicologic Pathology. Washington, STP/ARP/AFIP, 1995, URG-1, 1–19.
35 Hirose M, Imaida K, Ito H, Hayashi M, Ishihara Y, Ito N: Effects of chloroform and dimethylnitrosamine in renal carcinogenesis in unilaterally nephrectomized rats fed formic acid 2-[4-(5-nitro-2-furyl]-2-[thiazolyl]hydrazide. Carcinogenesis 1981;2:703–708.
36 Nogueira E: Rat renal carcinogenesis after chronic simultaneous exposure to lead acetate and N-nitrosodiethylamine. Virchows Arch B Cell Pathol 1987;53:365–374.
37 Bannasch P, Zerban H: Preneoplastic and neoplastic lesions of the kidney of the rat; in Bannasch P, Gössner W (eds): Pathology of Neoplasia and Preneoplasia in Rodents. EULEP Color Atlas. Stuttgart, Schattauer, 1994, pp 82–107.
38 Delahunt B, Wakefield J: Ultrastructure of streptozotocin-induced renal tumors in mice. Virchows Arch 1997;430:173–180.
39 Störkel S, Pannen B, Thoenes W, Steart PV, Wagner S, Drenckhahn D: Intercalated cells as a probable source for the development of renal oncocytoma. Virchows Arch B Cell Pathol 1988;56: 185–189.
40 Störkel S, Steart PV, Drenckhahn D, Thoenes W: The human chromophobe cell renal carcinoma – Its probable relation to intercalated cells of the collecting duct. Virchows Arch B Cell Pathol 1988;56:237–245.
41 Ito N: Experimental studies on tumors of the urinary system of rats induced by chemical carcinogens. Acta Pathol Jpn 1973;23:87–109.
42 Hard GC: Tumors of the kidney, renal pelvis and ureter. IARC Sci Publ 1976;6:73–101.
43 Mao P, Molnar JJ: The fine structure and histochemistry of lead-induced renal tumors in rats. Am J Pathol 1967;50:571–603.
44 Hard GC, Butler WH: Ultrastructural aspects of renal adenocarcinoma induced in the rat by dimethylnitrosamine. Cancer Res 1971;31:336–372.
45 Hard GC, Butler WH: Morphogenesis of epithelial neoplasms induced in the rat kidney by dimethylnitrosamine. Cancer Res 1971;31:1496–1505.
46 McGiven AR, Ireton HJ: Renal epithelial dysplasia and neoplasia in rats given dimethylnitrosamine. J Pathol 1972;108:187–190.
47 Hruban Z, Mochizuki Y, Morris HP, Slesers A: Ultrastructure of Morris renal tumors. J Natl Cancer Inst 1973;50:1487–1495.
48 Merkow LP, Epstein SM, Slifkin M, Pardo M: The ultrastructure of renal neoplasms induced by aflatoxin B1. Cancer Res 1975;33:1608–1614.

49 Gusek W: The ultrastructure of cycasin-induced adenomas of kidney. Virchows Arch A Pathol Anat Histol 1975;365:221–237.
50 Dees JH, Reuber MD, Trump BF: Adenocarcinoma of the kidney. I. Ultrastructure of renal adenocarcinomas induced by rats by (N-(4′-fluoro-4-biphenylyl)acetamide. J Natl Cancer Inst 1976; 57:779–794.
51 Brummer C, Rabes HM: Morphology and proliferation kinetics of early tumor stages induced by dimethylnitrosamine in rat kidneys. Virchows Arch B Cell Pathol 1992;62:133–142.
52 Bannasch P, Nogueira E, Zerban H: Zytologie und Zytogenese experimenteller epithelialer Nierentumoren. Verh Dtsch Ges Pathol 1989;73:301–313.
53 Hull MT, Eble JN: Myelinoid lamellated cytoplasmic inclusions in human renal adenocarcinomas: An ultrastructural study. Ultrastruct Pathol 1987;12:41–48.
54 Nogueira E, Klimek F, Weber E, Bannasch P: Origin of rat renal clear cell tumors from the collecting duct. Virchows Arch B Cell Pathol 1989;57:275–283.
55 Ahn YS, Zerban H, Grobholz R, Bannasch P: Sequential changes in glycogen content, expression of glucose transporters and enzymic patterns during development of clear/acidophilic cell tumors in rat kidney. Carcinogenesis 1992;13:2329–2334.
56 Eble JN (ed): Tumors and Tumor-Like Conditions of the Kidneys and Ureters. New York, Churchill Livingstone, 1990.
57 Oberling CH, Rivière M, Haguenau F: Ultrastructure of clear cells in renal carcinoma and its importance for the demonstration of their renal origin. Nature 1960;186:402–403.
58 Tannenbaum M: Ultrastructural pathology of human renal cell tumors. Pathol Annu 1971;6:249–277.
59 Shiao YH, Rice JM, Anderson LM, Diwan BA, Hard GC: von Hippel-Lindau gene mutations in N-nitrosodimethylamine-induced rat renal epithelial tumors. J Natl Cancer Inst 1998;90:1720–1723.
60 Ibrahim RE, Weinberg DS, Weidner N: Atypical cysts and carcinomas of the kidneys in the phacomatoses. Cancer 1989;63:148–157.
61 Nogueira E, Bannasch P: Cellular origin of rat renal oncocytoma. Lab Invest 1988;59:337–343.
62 Hamperl H: Onkocyten und Onkocytome. Virchows Arch A Pathol Anat 1962;355:452–483.
63 van der Walt JD, Reid HAS, Risdon RA, Shaw HF: Renal oncocytoma. A review of the literature and report of an unusual multicentric case. Virchows Arch A Pathol Anat Histol 1983;398:291–304.
64 Chang A, Harawi SJ: Oncocytes, oncocytosis, and oncocytic tumors. Pathol Annu 1992;27:263–304.
65 Krech R, Zerban H, Bannasch P: Mitochondrial anomalies in renal oncocytes induced in rat by N-nitrosomorpholine. Eur J Cell Biol 1981;25:331–339.
66 Tsuda H, Hacker HJ, Katayama H, Masui T, Ito N, Bannasch P: Correlative histochemical studies on preneoplastic and neoplastic lesions in the kidney of rats treated with nitrosamines. Virchows Arch B Cell Pathol 1986;51:385–404.
67 Zerban H, Nogueira E, Riedasch G, Bannasch P: Renal oncocytoma: Origin from the collecting duct. Virchows Arch B Cell Pathol 1987;52:375–387.
68 Ortmann M, Vierbuchen M, Fischer R: Renal oncocytoma. II. Lectin and immunohistochemical features indicating an origin from the collecting duct. Virchows Arch B Cell Pathol 1988;56:175–184.
69 Eble JN, Hull MT: Glycoconjugate expression in human renal oncocytomas. A lectin histochemical study. Arch Pathol Lab Med 1988;112:805–808.
70 Klein MJ, Valensi QJ: Proximal tubular adenoma of kidney with so-called oncocytic features. A clinicopathologic study of 13 cases of a rarely reported neoplasm. Cancer 1976;38:906–914.
71 Zollinger HU: Durch chronische Bleivergiftung erzeugte Nierenadenome und -carcinome bei Ratten und ihre Beziehung zu den entsprechenden Neubildungen des Menschen. Virchows Arch 1953;323: 694–710.
72 Rosen VR Jr, Castanera TJ, Kimmeldorf DJ, Jones DC: Renal neoplasms in the irradiated and nonirradiated Sprague-Dawley rat. Am J Pathol 1961;38:359–369.
73 Berdjis CC: Kidney tumours and irradiation pathogenesis of kidney tumours in irradiated rats. Oncologia (Basel) 1963;16:312–324.
74 Hiasa Y, Kitahori Y, Konishi N, Enoki N, Shimovama T, Miyashiro A: Trisodium nitrilotriacetate monohydrate: Promoting effects on the development of renal tubular cell tumors in rats treated with N-ethyl-N-hydroxy-ethylnitrosamine. J Natl Cancer Inst 1984;72:483–489.

75 Shirai T, Oshima M, Masuda A, Tamano S, Ito N: Promotion of 2-(ethylnitrosamino)ethanol-induced carcinogenesis in rats by nephrotoxic compounds: Positive responses with folic acid, basic lead acetate, and N-(3,5-dichlorophenyl)succinimide but not with 2,3-dibromo-i-propanol phosphate. J Natl Cancer Inst 1984;72:477–482.
76 Tanner DC, Lipsky M: Effect of lead acetate on N-(4-fluoro-4′-biphenyl)acetamide-induced renal carcinogenesis in the rat. Carcinogenesis 1984;5:1109–1113.
77 Alden CL, Kanerva RL: The pathogenesis of renal cortical tumors in rats fed 2% trisodium nitrilotriacetate monohydrate. Food Chem Toxicol 1982;20:441–450.
78 Alden CL, Kanerva RL: Reversibility of renal cortical lesions induced in rats by high doses of nitriloacetate in chronic feeding study. Food Chem Toxicol 1982;20:935–937.
79 Anderson RL, Alden CL, Merski JA: The effects of nitrilotriacetate on cation disposition and urinary tract toxicity. Food Chem Toxicol 1982;20:105–122.
80 Swenberg JA, Short B, Borhoff S, Strasser J, Charbonneau M: The comparative pathobiology of α_{2u}-globulin nephropathy. Toxicol Appl Pharmacol 1989;97:35–46.
81 Bannasch P, Mayer D, Krech R: Neoplastische und präneoplastische Veränderungen bei Ratten nach einmaliger oraler Applikation von N-Nitrosomorpholin. J Cancer Res Clin Oncol 1979;94: 233–248.
82 Holm-Nielsen P, Olsen TS: Ultrastructure of renal adenoma. Ultrastruct Pathol 1988;12:27–40.
83 Cohen C, McCue PA, Derose PB: Histogenesis of renal cell carcinoma and renal oncocytoma. An immunohistochemical study. Cancer 1988;62:1946–1951.
84 Bannasch P, Hacker HJ, Tsuda H, Zerban H: Aberrant regulation of carbohydrate metabolism and metamorphosis during renal carcinogenesis. Adv Enzyme Regul 1986;25:279–296.
85 Weber G: Enzymic programs in human renal adenocarcinomas; in Sufrin G, Beckley SA (eds): Renal Adenocarcinomas. Geneva, International Union Against Cancer, 1980, pp 45–50.
86 Mayer D, Bannasch P: Activity of glycogen synthase and phosphorylase and glucose-6-phosphate content in renal clear cell carcinomas. J Cancer Res Clin Oncol 1988;114:369–372.
87 Steinberg P, Störkel S, Oesch F, Thoenes W: Carbohydrate metabolism in human renal clear cell carcinoma. Lab Invest 1992;67:506–511.
88 Bannasch P: Pathogenesis of hepatocellular carcinoma: Sequential cellular, molecular, and metabolic changes; in Boyer JL, Ockner RK (eds): Progress in Liver Diseases. Philadelphia, Saunders, 1996, pp 161–197.
89 Bannasch P, Klimek F, Mayer D: Early bioenergetic changes in hepatocarcinogenesis: Preneoplastic phenotypes mimic responses to insulin and thyroid hormone. J Bioenerget Biomemb 1997;29: 303–313.
90 Nehrbass D, Klimek F, Bannasch P: Overexpression of insulin receptor substrate-1 emerges early in hepatocarcinogenesis and elicits preneoplastic hepatic glycogenosis. Am J Pathol 1998;152:341–345.
91 Kellerer M, von Eye Corleta H, Mühlhöfer A, Capp E, Mosthaf L, Bock S, Petrides PE, Häring HU: Insulin- and insulin-like growth-factor-I receptor tyrosine-kinase activities in human renal carcinoma. Int J Cancer 1995;62:501–507.
92 Oka H, Chatani Y, Hoshino R, Ogawa O, Kakehi Y, Terachi T, Okada Y, Kawaichi M, Kohno M, Yoshida O: Constitutive activation of mitogen-activated protein (MAP) kinases in human renal cell carcinoma. Cancer Res 1995;55:4182–4187.
93 Heatfield BM, Hinton DE, Trump BF: Adenocarcinoma of the kidney. II. Enzyme histochemistry of renal adenocarcinomas induced in rats by N-(4-fluoro-4-biphenylyl)acetamide. J Natl Cancer Inst 1976;57:795–808.
94 Ohmori T, Hiasa Y, Murata Y, Williams GM: Gamma glutamyl transpeptidase activity in carcinogen-induced epithelial lesions of the rat kidney. Gann 1982;73:543–548.
95 Tsuda H, Moore MA, Asamoto M, Inoue T, Fukushima S, Ito N, Satoh K, Amelizad Z, Oesch F: Immunohistochemically demonstrated altered expression of cytochrome P-450 molecular forms and epoxide hydrolase in N-ethyl-N-hydroxyethylnitrosamine-induced rat kidney and liver lesions. Carcinogenesis 1987;8:711–717.
96 Ahn YS, Zerban H, Bannasch P: Expression of glucose transporter isoforms (GLUT1, GLUT2) and activities of hexokinase, pyruvate kinase and malic enzyme in preneoplastic and neoplastic rat renal basophilic cell lesions. Virchows Arch B Cell Pathol 1993;63:351–357.

97 Tsuda H, Moore MA, Asamoto M, Satoh K, Tsuchida S, Sato K, Ichihara A, Ito N: Comparison of the various forms of glutathione S-transferase with glucose-6-phosphate dehydrogenase and gamma-glutamyl transpeptidase as markers of preneoplastic and neoplastic lesions in rat kidney induced by N-ethyl-N-hydroxyethylnitrosamine. Jpn J Cancer Res 1985;76:919–929.
98 Mayer D, Weber E, Kadenbach B, Bannasch P: Immunocytochemical demonstration of cytochrome-c-oxidase as a marker for renal oncocytes and oncocytomas. Toxicol Pathol 1989;17:46–49.
99 Ahn YS, Rempel A, Zerban H, Bannasch P: Over-expression of glucose transporter isoform GLUT1 and hexokinase I in rat renal oncocytic tubules and oncocytomas. Virchows Arch B Cell Pathol 1994;425:63–68.
100 Fischer R: Über den histochemischen Nachweis oxydativer Enzyme in Onkozyten verschiedener Organe. Virchows Arch Pathol Anat Physiol Klin Med 1961;334:445–452.
101 Tandler B, Shipkey FH: Ultrastructure of Warthin's tumor. I. Mitochondria. J Ultrastruct Res 1964;11:292–305.
102 Walker C, Everitt J, Freed JJ, Knudson AG Jr, Whiteley LO: Altered expression of transforming growth factor-alpha in hereditary rat renal cell carcinoma. Cancer Res 1991;51:2973–2978.
103 Deguchi J, Kawabata T, Kondo A, Okada S: Transforming growth factor-alpha expression of renal proximal tubules in Wistar rats treated with ferric and aluminium nitrilotriacetate. Jpn J Cancer Res 1993;84:649–655.
104 Erlandsson R: Molecular genetics of renal cell carcinoma. Cancer Genet Cytogenet 1998;104:1–18.
105 Nicoll JW, Swann PF, Pegg AE: Effect of dimethylnitrosamine on persistence of methylated guanines in rat liver and kidney DNA. Nature 1975;254:261–262.
106 Singer B: N-Nitroso alkylating agents: Formation and persistence of alkyl derivatives in mammalian nucleic acids as contributing factors in carcinogenesis. J Natl Cancer Inst 1979;62:1329–1339.
107 Toyokuni S, Sagripanti JL: DNA single- and double-strand breaks produced by ferric nitrilotriacetate in relation to renal tubular carcinogenesis. Carcinogenesis 1993;14:223–227.
108 Toyokuni S, Mori T, Dizdaroglu M: DNA base modifications in renal chromatin of Wistar rats treated with a renal carcinogen, ferric nitrilotriacetate. Int J Cancer 1994;57:123–128.
109 Umemura T, Sai K, Takagi A, Hasegawa R, Kurokawa Y: Oxidative DNA damage, lipid peroxidation and nephrotoxicity induced in the rat kidney after ferric nitrilotriacetate administration. Cancer Lett 1990;54:95–100.
110 Toyokuni S, Uchida K, Okamoto K, Hattori-Nakakuki Y, Hiai H, Stadtman ER: Formation of 4-hydroxy-2-nonenal-modified proteins in the renal proximal tubules of rats treated with a renal carcinogen, ferric nitriloacetate. Proc Natl Acad Sci USA 1994;91:2616–2620.
111 Sai K, Takagi A, Umemura T, Hasegawa R, Kurokawa Y: Relation of 8-hydroxydeoxyguanosine formation in rat kidney to lipid peroxidation, glutathione level and relative organ weight after a single administration of potassium bromate. Jpn J Cancer Res 1991;82:165–169.
112 Kasai H, Nishimura S, Kurokawa Y, Hayashi Y: Oral administration of the renal carcinogen, potassium bromate, specifically produces 8-hydroxydeoxyguanosine in rat target organ DNA. Carcinogenesis 1987;8:1959–1961.
113 Decker HJ, Weidt EJ, Brieger J: The von Hippel-Lindau tumor suppressor gene. A rare and intriguing disease opening new insight into basic mechanisms of carcinogenesis. Cancer Genet Cytogenet 1996; 93:74–83.
114 Kikuchi Y, Kobayashi E, Nishizawa M, Hamazaki S, Okuda S, Hino O: Cloning of the rat homologue of the von Hippel-Lindau tumor suppressor gene and its nonsomatic mutation in rat renal cell carcinomas. Jpn J Cancer Res 1995;86:905–909.
115 Walker C, Ahn Y-T, Everitt J, Yuan X: Renal cell carcinoma development in the rat independent of alterations at the VHL gene locus. Mol Carcinog 1996;15:154–161.
116 Shiao YH, Diwan BA, Perantoni AO, Calvert RJ, Zbar B, Lerman MI, Rice JM: Polymerase chain reaction-single-strand conformation polymorphism analysis for the VHL gene in chemically induced kidney tumors of rats using intron-derived primers. Mol Carcinog 1997;19:230–235.
117 Matsumoto K, Tsuda H, Iwase T, Ito M, Nishida Y, Oyama F, Titani K, Ushijima T, Nagao M, Hirono I: Absence of ras family point mutations at codons 12, 13 and 61 in N-ethyl-N-hydroxyethylnitrosamine- or N-nitrosomorpholine-induced renal cell tumors in rats. Jpn J Cancer Res 1992;83:933–936.

118 Everitt JI, Goldsworthy TL, Wolf DS, Walker CL: Hereditary renal cell carcinoma in the Eker rat: A rodent familial cancer syndrome. J Urol 1992;148:1932–1936.
119 Hino O, Mitani H, Nishizawa M, Katsuyama H, Kobayashi E, Hirayama Y: A novel renal cell carcinoma susceptibility gene maps on chromosome 10 in the Eker rat. Jpn J Cancer Res 1993;84: 1106–1109.
120 Eker R, Mossige J, Johannessen JV, Aars H: Hereditary renal adenomas and adenocarcinomas in rats. Diagn Histopathol 1981;4:99–110.
121 Walker C, Goldsworthy TL, Wolf D, Everitt J: Predisposition to renal cell carcinoma due to alteration of a cancer susceptibility gene. Science 1992;255:1693–1695.
122 Yeung RS, Buetow KH, Testa JR, Knudson AG: Susceptibility to renal carcinoma in the Eker rat involves a tumor suppressor gene on chromosome 10. Proc Natl Acad Sci USA 1993;90:8038–8042.
123 Hino O, Kobayashi T, Tsuchiya H, Kikuchi Y, Kobayashi E, Mitani H, Hirayama Y: The predisposing gene of the Eker rat inherited cancer syndrome is tightly linked to the tuberous sclerosis (TSC2) gene. Biochem Biophys Res Commun 1994;203:1302–1308.
124 Kobayashi T, Hirayama Y, Kobayashi E, Kubo Y, Hino O: A germline insertion in the tuberous sclerosis (Tsc2) gene gives rise to the Eker rat model of dominantly inherited cancer. Nat Genet 1995;9:70–75.
125 Kubo Y, Mitani H, Hino O: Allelic loss at the predisposing gene locus in spontaneous and chemically induced renal cell carcinomas in the Eker rat. Cancer Res 1994;54:2633–2635.
126 Kubo Y, Klimek F, Kikuchi Y, Bannasch P, Hino O: Early detection of Knudson's two-hits in preneoplastic renal cells of the Eker rat model by the laser microdissection procedure. Cancer Res 1995;55:989–990.
127 Jin F, Wienecke R, Xiao G-H, Maize JC, Declue JE, Yeung RS: Suppression of tumorigenicity by the wild-type tuberous sclerosis 2 (Tsc2) gene and its C-terminal region. Proc Natl Acad Sci USA 1996;93:9154–9159.
128 Orimoto K, Tsuchiya H, Kobayasi T, Matsuda T, Hino O: Suppression of the neoplastic phenotype by replacement of the Tsc2 gene in Eker rat renal carcinoma cells. Biochem Biophys Res Commun 1996;219:70–75.
129 Kobayashi T, Mitani H, Takahashi R-I, Hirabayashi M, Ueda M, Tamura H, Hino O: Transgenic rescue from embryonic lethality and renal carcinogenesis in the Eker rat model by introduction of a wild-type Tsc2 gene. Proc Natl Acad Sci USA 1997;94:3990–3993.
130 Kobayashi T, Urakami S, Hirayama Y, Yamamoto T, Nishizawa M, Takahara T, Kubo Y, Hino O: Intragenic Tsc2 somatic mutations as Knudson's second hit in spontaneous and chemically induced renal carcinomas in the Eker rat model. Jpn J Cancer Res 1997;88:254–261.
131 Urakami S, Tokuzen R, Tsuda H, Igawa M, Hino O: Somatic mutation of the tuberous sclerosis (Tsc2) tumor suppressor gene in chemically induced rat renal carcinoma cell. J Urol 1997;158:275–278.
132 Satake N, Urakami S, Hirayama Y, Izumi K, Hino O: Biallelic mutations of the Tsc2 gene in chemically induced rat renal cell carcinoma. Int J Cancer 1998;77:895–900.
133 Wienecke R, König A, Declue JE: Identification of tuberin, the tuberous sclerosis-2 product. J Biol Chem 1995;270:16409–16414.
134 Xiao G-H, Shoarinejad F, Jin F, Golemis EA, Yeung RS: The tuberous sclerosis 2 gene product, tuberin, functions as a Rab5 GTPase activating protein (GAP) in modulating endocytosis. J Biol Chem 1997;272:6097–6100.
135 Tsuchiya H, Orimoto K, Kobayashi T, Hino O: Presence of potent transcriptional activation domains in the predisposing tuberous sclerosis (Tsc2) gene product of the Eker rat model. Cancer Res 1996; 56:429–433.
136 Orimoto K, Tsuchiya H, Sakurai J, Nishizawa M, Hino O: Identification of cDNAs induced by the tumor suppressor Tsc2 gene using a conditional expression system in Tsc2 mutant (Eker) rat renal carcinoma cells. Biochem Biophys Res Commun 1998;247:728–733.

Prof. Dr. P. Bannasch, Abteilung für Cytopathologie (C0100), Deutsches Krebsforschungszentrum, Im Neuenheimer Feld 280, D–69120 Heidelberg (Germany)
Tel. +49 6221 423202, Fax +49 6221 423222, E-Mail p.bannasch@dkfz-Heidelberg.de

Author Index

Subject Index